THE
Great Ormond Street Nurse

My Life as a Student Nurse in the 1960s

THE
Great Ormond Street Nurse

My Life as a Student Nurse in the 1960s

Vanessa Martin

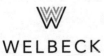

WELBECK

Published by Welbeck
An imprint of Welbeck Non-Fiction Limited,
part of Welbeck Publishing Group.
Based in London and Sydney.

Published by Welbeck in 2022

A CIP catalogue record for this book is available from the British Library

ISBN
Paperback – 9781787399105
eBook – 9781787399549

Typeset by Roger Walker
Printed in Great Britain by CPI Books, Chatham, Kent

10 9 8 7 6 5 4 3 2 1

The Forest Stewardship Council® is an international
nongovernmental organisation that promotes environmentally
appropriate, socially beneficial, and economically viable management
of the world's forests. To learn more, visit www.fsc.org

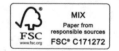

www.welbeckpublishing.com

*To my two sons, Jonathan and James,
and my daughter Philippa, who joined me
during this time.*

CONTENTS

PROLOGUE

"Nurse, did you wipe the thermometer before you put it under that child's arm?"

Nurse? That was me. My heart jumped and I swallowed a gasp. No, no, please no.

I turned around and was mortified to find Matron standing behind me, alongside the ward sister.

"No, Matron," I replied meekly, my neck hot under the starched white collar of my uniform.

"Go down to my office now and wait for me there," Matron ordered.

I didn't have to be asked twice.

I was nine weeks into my training and I had just left preliminary training school (PTS) at the Hospital for Sick Children, Great Ormond Street, known then as GOS. This was my first day on the ward. I'd been nervous but excited as I put on my uniform early that morning.

The pink-and-white striped cotton dress was comfortable, though utterly shapeless. Why had we ever complained about school uniforms? They were the height of fashion compared to these. But the candy-striped dresses were practical – except for the wretched starched white collars, which rubbed like anything. There were pockets for everything, from spare safety nappy pins to a pen torch and

1

notebook. Then there were the black stockings, the seams of which *had* to be straight. And no make-up or jewellery. All topped off with my GOS first-year nurse's cap.

I felt really proud. It was 1962, the NHS was in its second decade, and I was part of it, a student nurse at London's world-renowned children's hospital. But now, just a few hours later, I was already in trouble.

Matron's office. What on earth was she going to say to me?

I trudged down the corridor, the squeak of my sensible black lace-up shoes barely noticeable above the rush of blood in my head, and waited outside her office. I felt nauseous and cross with myself, anxious about the dressing-down I was no doubt about to receive. Why was this happening? Last thing I knew, a third-year student was handing me a thermometer in a pot of Hycolin disinfectant, telling me to take a particular child's temperature.

"Should I not dry the thermometer?" I'd asked her.

She sighed, clearly not liking this impertinent first year questioning her. Her special Great Ormond Street strings cap – shaped like an inverted ice cream cone – might just as well have been a Belisha beacon, announcing loudly and clearly her seniority over me. "You're not in PTS now," she snapped. "You're working on the real wards."

So, I duly did as I was told. I took the pot to the bedside of the little boy in question, endeavouring to dry the thermometer as best I could using my fingers, and shook down the mercury to its lowest point. I put the thermometer under his arm, focused on the job at hand, and didn't hear the soon-to-be familiar footsteps come to a stop behind me. Matron.

And here Matron was now, striding towards me as I waited like a naughty schoolgirl outside the headmistress's office. Gulp.

This wasn't the first time I'd met Matron. Miss Gwendoline Kirby had interviewed me over two years earlier, when I had just started at sixth form. I was actually surprisingly relaxed that day; Matron put me at ease and asked questions I'd prepared for. Why did I wish to train for this profession? Why should they choose me? Could I be relied on to complete the course? After a second interview with Matron's deputy, at which I was asked similar questions, I was told to sit in the waiting room. Fortunately, it wasn't long before I was informed that I'd been accepted. It had all, surprisingly perhaps, gone to plan.

Now was a different story. Did Matron regret her faith in me?

"Well, Nurse Owen. Would you like to explain why you took a child's temperature without drying the thermometer? What have you been taught in training?"

I knew exactly what we'd been taught in training. I also realised the third-year nurse had dropped me in it. She'd probably seen Matron coming, when my back was turned and panicked, knowing Matron would inspect the child's observation chart at the end of his bed and see that the temperature was overdue. She'd shoved the thermometer pot into my hand and ordered me to do the job.

Since she was my senior, I just did as I was told. This was infuriating and so unfair. I would *never* grab a thermometer in a pot without the tray. How else could you clean and dry it? And if I'd been in her clumpy lace-up shoes, I'd have gone to the boy myself and taken his temperature, not passed the thermometer incorrectly to a novice student on her first day. If Matron asked me why the temperature was being taken late, I'd have given her my reason.

"Nurse?" Matron held firm eye contact with me, keen to hear my answer.

"Never take a thermometer in a pot of Hycolin without the thermometer tray," I replied to her question.

"And why is that necessary, Nurse?"

"So that you can dry the thermometer, Matron."

"And what might be caused by Hycolin coming into contact with a child's skin?"

"It can cause redness, and irritation to the skin."

"Yes, Nurse." She nodded, eyes down at her desk while she made some notes, before focusing all her attention on me so that I felt as small as one of the children on the ward. "This might be your first day, Nurse Owen, but I expect better of you."

I thought about telling Matron what happened. That it wasn't my fault. After all, why should I take the blame? But there was no point moaning. I wasn't a grass, and I knew the hospital motto – "Children First and Always".

"I'm sorry, Matron. It won't happen again."

I'd make sure of that.

EARLY YEARS

I was born in 1944 in London. My father was in the South African forces and had to return to South Africa after the war. I lived with my mother and grandmother in my grandmother's house in Barnes, southwest London. I was very fond of my grandmother, who was Victorian in her ways and determined to bring me up to be a lady. Some of my earliest memories, before I started school, are of Derry & Toms, the large department store on Kensington High Street, where my grandmother occasionally took me for tea.

Derry & Toms was renowned for its enormous roof garden, created at great expense, with tons of soil and hundreds of shrubs and large mature trees craned onto the roof. There was even a duck pond and a flowing stream, home to a flock of exotic pink flamingos.[1]

The roof garden had an outdoor restaurant with round tables and white parasols with blue trimming, where it was very fashionable to have tea. My grandmother would take me by taxi, then up in the store's private lift to the roof garden, where we'd be shown to our pre-booked table for two.

Here, she was determined to teach me my manners. I had to keep my hands in my lap and never put my arm or elbows on the table. I had to dab my mouth with the napkin, not wipe it. I had to hold my china cup daintily with three fingers, never a fist, and I had to "show" my sandwiches and cakes to my plate before eating them. It was the height of sophistication – literally 100 feet above street level.

I was nine when my father returned from South Africa. For that first year, I was sent to a convent boarding school, where I missed home desperately. The only thing I enjoyed was learning to ride on a horse called Silver, whose horseshoe I still prize. I remember a list being produced that allocated us a bathroom for our weekly bath.

I never bathed properly unless I was allocated the "green bathroom". This was small and modern with a plastic bath that was familiar to me. I'd always been nervous of the noises from the overhead plumbing in public lavatories and all the other bathrooms at the convent had metal baths that echoed when filled and emptied. The worst of them all was the "white bathroom". Its bath was huge and sat on a platform with steps up to it. Water rushed from a large mixer tap and thundered into the metal bath.

When I was allocated the white bathroom, I had a system for coping with my terror. As soon as the nun had filled the bath and left, I'd sit on the floor as far away from the bath as I dared until I heard her return. Then I would rush up the steps and jump into the end farthest from the taps and pretend I'd just finished washing. I never knew why she didn't notice how clean the water was when she pulled the plug.

My mother brought me home after a year when she realised just how unhappy I was. She and my father had moved to a small flat in Clapham. She was having a baby and wanted me to be there when he was born. My brother, John, arrived not long after I returned home.

I was sent to the local primary school in Clapham for a short time, where I met a lovely girl called Jackie Stone and we became great friends. I remember our gifted maths teacher teaching us that "14 Jacqueline pounds makes one Jaqueline Stone", which we found hilarious. Jackie remembers our P.E. kit. We wore vests tucked into dark green knickers that had a pocket for our hankie!

Around this time, my family and I returned to live with my grandmother, so I had to commute into Clapham by walking across Hammersmith Bridge to catch the trolley bus. The trolleys had two booms attached to their roof. These hooked onto the overhead lines to power them. Sometimes one of these booms would detach from the line and the conductor had to remove the long pole that lived under the bus and hook the boom back onto the line. The school was appropriately tolerant of my occasional lateness; the notorious trolleys were somewhat infamous for being fickle.

After my 11-plus exam, I was fortunate enough to be offered a place in a new girls' school being built in New Malden. For the first year, there were only two classes of 30 pupils each and we were to be taught in Portacabins with a full quota of staff until the school itself was ready to be opened. Gillian, Maria, Susan and I travelled together and made the lengthy 72 bus journey every day. We met each morning at the back of the top of the bus for the journey and returned together each evening.

As younger pupils joined the school, it was very strange for us always to be the most senior pupils and the most privileged. It was there that I met my friend Carol, with whom occasionally I would stay overnight. She had three brothers, and although by then I had a baby brother of my own, the chaos in her house was quite new to me. There was no peace where she lived as the boys somersaulted from chair to chair in the living room and were constantly under your feet. I even found the youngest in my room, hiding under the curtain of my dressing table when I was about to undress to go to bed. Carol soon gave him short shrift, but all I had suffered was a fright.

I had wanted to work with children since I was a teenager. I spent some of my school holidays volunteering in both an old people's home and in a day nursery. Although I found working with the elderly rewarding, it was the children who fascinated me. I had a rapport with them. One day on my return from the nursery, I regaled my mother with tales of the little children. She listened carefully, asking me questions. I could tell she was considering something and wondered what she was going to say.

"Vanessa, you clearly like working with children. You've always been practical and caring, and you're good at looking after your brother. Why don't you apply to the Hospital for Sick Children, Great Ormond Street?"

"Great Ormond Street?"

"It's a London hospital just for paediatrics. You can train there to be a registered sick children's nurse."

"I can?"

Before the war, my mother had trained as a physiotherapist at Guy's Hospital in London, just as physiotherapy was striving to become a profession in its own right.

"If I could be a physio, there's no reason you can't be a children's nurse."

I discussed my mother's suggestion of applying to GOS with my school headmistress. She wasn't as encouraging.

"You're an average student, Vanessa. You need five O-levels with good grades to be accepted at the hospital. Competition for a place will be too fierce. Have you considered anything else?"

No, I hadn't. My friend Carol had ambitions to become an air hostess. I was a little more grounded.

That night, I spoke to my mother.

"You've nothing to lose by trying," she said.

So, I did. I applied.

I was invited to an interview. Matron did question me on my mock examination results as I was still waiting for my official O-level results. She was particularly interested in my maths. Calculating the dosage of medicines to be given to children could be challenging, and a mistake could be disastrous. Matron was pleased that I had done well in the subject and I hoped to get a good grade when I received my results the next month.

After my second interview with the deputy matron, I was thrilled to find that I was being offered a place at Great Ormond Street Hospital and would begin my training in September 1962. It wasn't until many years later that I came across an article in the *Nurses' League Journal*. A member of the July 1957 intake which we called a 'set' recalled how Miss Kirby told her during her interview that she normally had 1,000 applicants a year applying to train at GOS but could only accept 120 (four intakes of 30 students per year). Miss Kirby's comment to this 17-year-old girl was, "So what do you think I can do for you?" No wonder my headmistress had been so negative about the likelihood of my being accepted for training.

One thing Matron did say after she had offered me my place was, "Miss Owen, rather than continuing with your A-Levels, I'd like you to have some work experience, preferably with children." She smiled while adding, "I suggest discussing this with your parents and your headmistress."

And this is where my headmistress surprised me. Once she discovered I'd been accepted at Great Ormond Street, she went out of her way to search for a suitable family for whom I could work as an au pair. She found a place through a relative of hers in Germany.

In 1961, I moved in with the Becker family to look after their three young children: Cristian who was five, Katrina who was three and Dinah who was nine months. They lived near Hamburg in a town on the Elbe called Geesthacht, famous for the dam that was built across the river not long before I arrived.

Daily life there was different from London. My routine included the general care of the children and household duties. In the mornings, unless it was raining, I would open the bedroom windows to air the bedding on the windowsills. Sometimes I'd be asked to go to the local shop for breakfast provisions. I'd collect lovely fresh croissants and fresh milk, which we collected in a small metal churn with a carrying handle. After breakfast I made the beds. Sometimes I'd hang out the washing, every garment meticulously pegged in order of size, smallest to biggest, so that the neighbours knew we were an organised household. When I did the ironing, this included all the underwear and towels.

The children kept me occupied for most of the day as they didn't go to nursery or school. Katrina always wanted to please and never made a fuss. The baby was delightful. Christian was a bright, intelligent boy. Every bedtime, I'd read to the two older children before they settled to sleep. Christian would always say, "You haven't done enough reading yet. You need to read another chapter to practise your German."

He was also quite protective of me. If I took him to buy food from the local shop, he would stop me outside. "Tell me what you are going to ask for." When I told him, he would either say, "that's okay," or he'd correct my German. When I came out of the shop, he'd tell me how well I'd done, if that was the case.

Frau Becker was very good at baking and made delicious German tarts. Cristian always wanted to be served his slice first.

"Damen vor Herren Christian, das ist 'Ladies before Gentlemen' in Englisch," I told him one time.

Days later, he and Katrina were in the bath. They would take turns to be the first out and dried so that the other could have extra time to play in the water. It was Christian's turn to get out first as he well knew. As I went to help him, he gave me a sly smile and said in perfect English, "Ladies before gentlemen." Despite his charm, he didn't get away with it.

After nine months, it was time to come home. I'd really enjoyed looking after all the children and I'd learnt basic German from them in return. But it was time for the next chapter in my life.

FIRST YEAR

I began my sick children's training in September 1962, along with 29 other young women from all over the country who would be in the same set as me. We arrived at the nurses' home, 37 Guildford Street, London, (now the site of the Institute of Child Health) with our luggage, black sensible shoes and black nylon stockings. Our luggage had to be left in the foyer for a porter to take to our rooms as no men were allowed beyond that point, not even our fathers.

We had tea together, parents and daughters, in the nurses' lounge, politely balancing cups and saucers and Lyons jam sandwich cake on our knees. Soon we had to say our goodbyes and leave our parents with Matron. No doubt she'd be putting their minds at rest. There was no time to be nervous or sad; we were immediately whisked off with the sister tutors to be shown around the Nurses' Training School.

During our formal introductions there, we were reminded of how we were the privileged few, training at such an auspicious hospital and that we would be expected to rise to the challenge. Then it was time to be measured for our uniforms by the seamstress from the hospital sewing room. Though I never visited the sewing room, they did an awful lot of work for us. They didn't make our uniforms, but they would alter them and mend anything that got torn. They made our soft, fitted, cotton hospital masks, which were worn once and then sent to the laundry (the hospital changed to supplying the horrible paper ones when I was in my fourth year). They also made the theatre gowns and a shroud for a child if it died.

As we were fitted with our uniforms, we were informed of the strict dress code. It was distinctive from other hospitals. Dress hems were to be 15 inches from the ground, hair wasn't allowed to touch the collar (we were threatened with wearing hair nets if it did), no make-up or jewellery was permitted, and caps had to be sewn up in the proper way. They came starched flat from the laundry. We were never to wear our uniform outside the hospital when we were on duty, but we were given wonderful thick woollen capes, navy on the outside and red on the inside, to wear when walking between regulation buildings. Our starched white aprons, changed daily, had crossover straps that were pinned inside the back of our pink-and-white striped belts. (In practice, we tended to tuck them into the back of the belt.)

It would be a while before we would wear the distinctive buckled belts of a registered nurse. That day seemed a very long way off to a class of excited young students. Meanwhile, we were given the task of sewing our name tags on our dresses and on 15 aprons so that they could be sent to the laundry and returned personally to each of us.

The nurses' home was attached by a corridor to the main hospital. The home was run by the warden, whom we mostly visited when we need replacement caps. She was also the one who issued passes if you wanted to stay out late. You'd then have to show this pass to the porter on the main hospital desk, who would allow you in through the hospital to the nurses' home. The warden's room overlooked the foyer, and she locked the outside doors at 10 o'clock every evening without fail. If we knew the porter and we'd forgotten to apply for a pass, they'd usually take pity on us and allow us through.

It could be exhausting to adhere to such strict rules; many of us were away from home for the first time in our lives and it was only natural to be hoping for new freedoms. Unfortunately for us, in 1962, being under 21 meant that the hospital and Matron had an almost legal guardianship over their trainee nurses. This wasn't a responsibility they took lightly.

Our first taste of hospital food was surprisingly good that night. We then went to our bedrooms, where our luggage was waiting for us. The room was basic, with a bed, wardrobe and sink, but I could see I'd be comfortable there. After unpacking, I spent the rest of the evening chatting with the girls in the adjacent rooms, fellow students in my set.

Over the coming weeks, we would become friends. There was Carol from Yorkshire and Julia, a local London girl, both of whom I keep up with still. Then there was Christine from Manchester, who left after six months because she felt so homesick and isolated and, though she has sadly died, her husband is still in contact with me.

As for Matron, she had a flat on the mezzanine floor of the nurses' home and we would occasionally meet her in the lift. The staff sick bay was on the same floor and run like a hospital ward, as I was soon to find out.

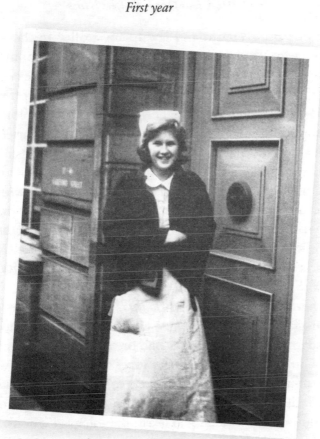

Me outside the nurses' home.

The School of Nursing was in a separate building, situated in Great Ormond Street on the east side of the hospital. There were classrooms with blackboards where medical staff came to teach us about their speciality. The school also had large practical rooms, containing beds and cots with dummy patients in them. There were trolleys and glass cupboards filled with all the instruments and solutions that were used on the wards. This set-up meant we could act out any scenario and lay up any trolley in the school that we would be asked for on the wards. These rooms were also used for practical finals exams when outside examiners would come in to test us. But this was a long way off yet.

Miss Eve Bendall had been appointed as senior sister tutor to the nursing school soon after we started our training. She had a calm and pleasant manner, and her approachability made her respected by all. She was always making sure we weren't having any problems with our practice on the wards. She'd regularly ask us individually if we had any problems with our training, reminding us that her door was always open. I never had an issue I wished to see her about, but it was reassuring to know I could go to her if need be. Interestingly, according to an appreciation of her in the *Nurses' League Journal* in 1971 after she left to take up a new post, her biggest concern was the retention of students – a topic that is even more concerning today.

Our nine weeks in preliminary training school was to introduce us to nursing and prepare us for our first ward. The tutors taught us the anatomy and physiology of the body, some of which I had learnt in biology at school. Now it was in much more depth and we had to understand and learn the differences in the adult anatomy and its function to that of a child's, which was different in many ways. Our lectures covered pregnancy and birth, and we had to learn the normal weights, lengths, head circumferences and their progressions, as well as the eruption of a baby's teeth.

The mental development of the child was another interesting subject. My mother had given birth to my baby sister, Maria, just two years before and I had been following her very closely. After these lectures, I went on a visit home and began listening more carefully to Maria's sentence formation, observing her sleeping pattern. I even took an interest in her toilet training. I came to the conclusion she was very forward for her age! Maria was behind with the number of teeth she had, which I now know is a family trait.

Routine care of the normal baby was another subject. Baby bathing, feeding, diet, nappy changing and care of the skin, hair and mouth. I remember us having large pots of zinc and caster-oil cream to put on babies' bottoms at every nappy change, which kept their skin in beautiful condition. Their learning through play was also an important subject.

We often worked in pairs. At first we practised the routine of bedmaking, which we would become so efficient at performing. We then went on to learn how to take temperatures under the arm for all young children so no child would bite on the mercury thermometer. We used the tray, which I failed to take to a child's bedside when Matron caught me on my first day. On it were six individual pots of Hycolin disinfectant, which contained the thermometers (one for each child in the ward). With them were two small bowls, one for clean cotton wool and the other for the dirty cotton wool after the thermometer was wiped.

While taking temperatures, we would find and count our companion's pulse, including the pulse in the neck, which was easier on babies. We would then discreetly try to count their respiration rate, which isn't easy to do, as patients' voluntary response is to change their breathing rate when they know you're counting it. Temperature, pulse and respiration rates were the main observations that gave an overall picture of the health of a child. Doing these observations with your student partner was amusing and often led to giggles as we all sat with thermometers in our armpits trying not to breathe.

Taking blood pressure readings took a lot more practice. Learning to pump up the cuff to just stop the radial pulse and not make the arm blue and painful, as well as getting the stethoscope the right way round so that you could hear the right changes in tone, was an art that took us a long time to master. We learnt the accurate recording of the results on charts that hung on the end of every bed – these were scrutinised by all staff. There was the taking of urine samples and testing it (usually our own). Thankfully, we were spared from taking stool (poo), vomit and sputum (spit) samples but learned the correct procedure, pots to put them in and the correct labelling. Then there was the giving of medicines and injections. The latter we practised into an orange rather than on each other.

The prevention of cross infection of bacteria and viruses was drummed into us before we were ready for the wards and we had to be competent in emergency care and resuscitation, which we practised on dummies. We had dummies of babies, young children and adults. We were tested on the different techniques needed to resuscitate all three. Saving the life of a child was essential for us to learn.

All these procedures were taken from our book of competencies provided by the General Nursing Council, the nursing regulation body. It was an exhausting nine weeks; there was so much to learn and remember for our exam, which we had to pass if we were to continue our training.

After we had taken this exam, about 12 of us were offered the opportunity to do a longer training course that was in the experimental stage. It involved spending a further year (our third year) in an adult training hospital, doing a combined training programme to qualify as a state registered nurse (SRN) and as a registered sick children's nurse (RSCN) in our fourth year. This would enable us to nurse adults as well as children. We chose the longer training, which I completed at Hammersmith Hospital.

Before we were sent on the wards, we had to pass a health check. This included having throat swabs taken. Mine came back positive to the haemolytic streptococcal bacteria, so I was immediately admitted to the sick bay on the mezzanine floor of the nurses' home and isolated. I was given intramuscular penicillin once every six hours in my backside for five days, which meant I missed being part of our set's official photograph for the hospital. Luckily, my new friends didn't forget me.

"Hey, Vanessa," I heard late one afternoon. The voice appeared to be coming from outside.

I got out of bed and peered out of my window, and there they were, huddled below on Guildford Street.

"Hello!" I waved. "What are you up to?"

"We're on our way back to the home. How are you feeling?"

"Perfectly well, thank you. I just wish I could get out of here and onto the ward, like you lot."

"Careful what you wish for," one of them joked. "We're exhausted and you've been in bed all day."

I sat in the window and we chatted for a bit. I was grateful that they kept me in the loop and was also madly envious that they'd made a start at nursing while I was stuck in the sick bay, a patient of all things – when I didn't even feel ill. I looked forward to their daily visits and counted down until my discharge, which eventually came following three clear throat swabs!

Following my discharge and clear throat swab results, I was allowed to begin working on my first ward as a "pinky nurse", which was what we were known as by other hospitals. My first shift hadn't exactly gone according to plan. There had been the thermometer incident. Four years later, at my final interview with Matron, she smilingly volunteered to remove it from my records. But this was a long way off. For now, it taught me a valuable lesson: to take responsibility for my own actions, even when others let you down.

Even then, I was part of a very old tradition. In the 1840s, Dr Charles West, supported by such visionaries as Charles Dickens, saw the opening of the first children's hospital in London at 49, Great Ormond Street. It began in 1852 in a seventeenth-century town house. Since then, its building has gone through many reincarnations. When the hospital first opened with 10 beds, it was intended for the poor children of the surrounding area: children who lived in squalid conditions, in filthy slums, with no sanitation, terrible diseases and a shockingly high level of infant mortality.[2/3]

It's hard now, looking back with twenty-first-century eyes, to believe that anyone would object to the building of a children's hospital, but there were fierce objections to it at the time. Many felt that children of the poor were expendable or that such a hospital would spread infectious diseases. Some feared that children born out of wedlock might be abandoned there, citing the example of the Foundling Hospital, a stone's throw away from Great Ormond Street. Nevertheless, the hospital grew.

By the time I arrived there in the 1960s, GOS was taking children from all over the country and even all over the world. Now in 2022 it still has a national and international reputation. But the ethos remains the same: to look after the health and wellbeing of children, to research into childhood diseases and treatments, and to train the medical profession in paediatrics.

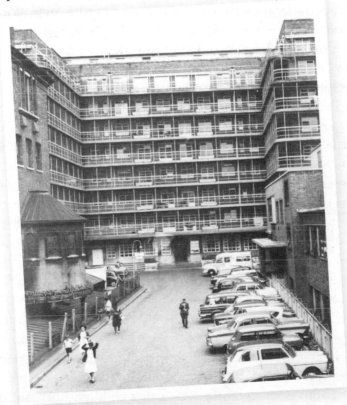

The Southwood building, c.1960 (Reprinted with permission, Archives Services, Great Ormond Street Hospital for Children NHS Foundation Trust)

Great Ormond Street Hospital was very different in my day to how it is today. In my time, the main entrance to the hospital was called the Southwood Entrance and was approached from Great Ormond Street. The hospital was divided into two main wings, with AB wards to the left and CD wards to the right of the building. All the wards had balconies where children could play in the fresh air. They were completely enclosed by metal grilles to keep our patients safe.

On the seventh floor was the private wing, which had its own lift. In fact, a few months before I started my training in February 1962, Prince Charles had his appendix removed there as an emergency. He was rushed by ambulance from Cheam School near Newbury and operated on by Mr David Waterson, staff surgeon. The 13-year-old heir to the throne declared, "I got here just in time before the thing exploded and was happily operated on and looked after by the nurses."[4]

WARD LIFE

It was now time for me to start working on my first ward, which was Ward 4C&D. This was a 20-bedded plastic surgery and eye ward where I would be for three months. I'd missed my first week on the ward and all my friends had settled in on theirs. I was nervous, but the registered nurses welcomed me. The ward sister, Sister O'Mara, was held in extremely high regard. She was an efficient and caring person who was passionate about the welfare of her students, always making sure we all had adequate breaks. Senior Staff Nurse Griffiths also graciously helped me settle in.

In those days, ward sisters ran the hospital with Matron at their head. They were all spinsters who had dedicated their lives to nursing, for which they were respected. The sister of each ward was very knowledgeable about all her patients' conditions and, as well as teaching us, was responsible for teaching and overseeing the work of the junior doctors, who had to have been registrars in an adult hospital before they were appointed to GOS.

Every weekday morning started with the main consultant's round. Before the round, the ward sister (or senior staff nurse), junior doctors, consultant and his registrar would have coffee together in the sister's office, discussing patients, operations, treatments and any problems they were having. When the ward round began, the ward sister would be the one who led it and had all the results of X-rays and blood tests to hand.

As first-year students, we were the bottom of the pile and weren't expected to join in the ward round. We did have to make sure that the children were on top of their beds and all their charts were complete and up to date. I remember once returning a child to bed as the "round" was approaching and being invited to stay. The consultant, who was doing some teaching with his staff, said, "Perhaps you too would like to learn a little more about this patient, Nurse?"

I looked at Sister, who beckoned for me to join the round, which I did. I felt honoured to have this opportunity.

We first years were mostly responsible for taking the routine observations of temperature, pulse and respirations (TPR) in the ward area. These were done once every four hours (sometimes more frequently) on every child and recorded on their chart. Because these charts hung on the end of every bed, they could be inspected by any member of staff, and we knew better than to *ever* forget to keep them updated.

Cleaning and sterilising were our daily morning chores and the sluice was our domain. This room was always filled with steam when the steriliser was boiling, and because everything was made of stainless steel, there was a lot of clanking when someone was working in there. Once the children were dressed and beds were made, we had to collect up the yellow enamel buckets of soiled nappies from the ward and take them to the sluice. The nappies would be put in a special bin and the buckets with their lids were put in the steriliser to be boiled along with the metal potties, utensils, bedpans and bottles.

The sluice was dominated by this large steriliser. It had a tap with a movable arm to fill it with water for the morning boil. It took so long to fill up the wretched thing that many a student left the water running while they did something else – which often resulted in flooding the sluice. News of this sort spread around the hospital very quickly, especially if water got through to the floor below.

Against the wall there were four vertical taps that turned upwards. If any naughty boys from the ward managed to get into the forbidden room, all hell would break loose. Turning on all four taps together would create a rainstorm, soaking the walls and the floor, and the boys loved the chaos. To prevent flooding to the floor below, we would rush in to turn off the taps and throw the dirty laundry on to the floor to soak up the water. We ourselves would get soaked. I remember doing this once wearing my strings cap (the one worn in our final year). Before Matron caught me with this limp rag on my head, I had to run across to the warden's office in the nurses' home for a new one, sewing it up with great speed before I could return to the ward.

Bedmaking was another important and repetitive chore carried out with military precision by the nurses. We'd practised it during training, but now this was for real. Actual children would sleep in these beds. It was done by two nurses because it was quicker in pairs.

All the bed linen had to have special hospital corners so that everything lay symmetrically. A strip of rubber and linen, called a draw sheet, was tucked across the middle of the bed for its child occupant to sit on so that, in the event of an accident, it would save staff having to change all the bed linen. Pillows were to have the open edges facing away from the door and bed wheels were to be facing inwards. This task was completed after breakfast in precision time, with all the children on the medical wards either sitting or lying on the draw sheet over their made bed, ready for the ward round.

The discipline of bedmaking harks back to Florence Nightingale's time as a nurse in the Crimean War, looking after wounded soldiers in the field and setting up a military hospital. Bedmaking is still of utmost importance in the military.

Jane Fryer of the *Daily Mail*[5] writes about army training at Sandhurst, where morning routine for the cadets begins in the bedroom. Hospital corners on their bed sheets are made as sharp as knives and the sheets are anchored to the bed frame beneath with bulldog clips. The closed ends of the pillowcases must always face the door. The general in command of the academy says that, "All of these skills can promote broader empowerment, self-discipline and leadership skills." The cadets confirm that rules such as these improve their confidence, self-belief and teamwork, and make them much more organised and better at decision-making.

Florence Nightingale went on to pioneer nurse training at St Thomas' Hospital and later advised on the setting up of the first specialist sick children's nurse training at GOS in 1878.[6] Evidence of this could still very much be seen on the wards where I trained and worked. When the importance of bedmaking was drummed into us, I couldn't help but think of not only Nurse Nightingale, but also of Frau Becker and her sheet-airing routine.

After that initial shaky start on my first shift, I found my stride and, although every day brought something new and challenging, I got used to the routines of hospital life. The children on the surgical wards were admitted for a minimum of two to three days. There was no day-case surgery then. It wasn't as noisy as one might imagine, as the children were either being prepared for theatre or being nursed after their operation so were either sedated or coming around from anaesthetics. Children were never left to cry.

On many of the medical wards, children were allowed to play, under supervision, with a toy car or a tricycle on the corridors. The wards were well ventilated as we had balconies on both sides. Unless it was winter or raining hard, the children could ride up and down the balconies too. We'd often carry a baby out there for fresh air or wheel out their cot. We'd also wheel out children in their beds if they were unable to walk. The ward nursery nurse would organise play for the children, mostly in the playroom, and a teacher might visit older bed-bound children if they were unable to attend the hospital school.

Life on the wards was so tiring. I didn't know if I would ever get used to it. Our working hours were long. On day duty, we worked a 48-hour week with one day off. We did one three-month stretch per year on night duty, working eight continuous nights of 12-hour shifts with four nights off. It was exhausting and isolating; we rarely saw anyone else and rarely had the same time off duty as those around us. One had a morning shift before a day off and a late shift after it, but it was sheer luck if a friend's shifts were the same as yours. We often used our time off to catch up on sleep.

Despite the exhausting work, there were many benefits to life at GOS. Not only did I get free meals and accommodation, but I also received a small salary that enabled me to be entirely independent from my family. At this time, young people were given apprenticeships to learn and obtain a qualification for a vocation like nursing, so we didn't have to apply for grants or look to our parents for support.

My treasured salary put down a deposit on a red Roberts Radio with my first wage, which brought me great joy between my draining shifts. A year later, I bought a tartan duffle coat from Marks & Spencer on Oxford Street. It still hangs in my wardrobe 58 years later, a lovely reminder of my first years of nursing.

On the night shift, our set was on shift together but on different wards with a different run of four nights off. This was the time when I might go home. I was envious of Julia, whose family lived just three stops on the Piccadilly line from Russell Square, the stop for GOS, which meant she could pop home for a few hours on her afternoons off.

I missed the comradeship and fun we had in preliminary training school and looked forward to our next block in the School of Nursing. As the hospital had a very hierarchical structure, it was rare to mix with anyone from another set, let alone another year. If Carol, Julia, Christine and I did meet up all together, it would have been at about 10 p.m., just before going to bed.

Our shifts started on the ward with a handover report in the sister's office given by the person who had taken charge of the previous shift. We would make notes in our

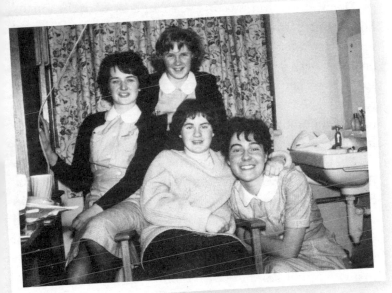

From left to right, Christine, me, Carol and Julia.

own notebook about changes in the patients' conditions, treatments and further care needed. At the end of this report, we would be allocated times for lunch or for our evening meal break so that we went to the dining room in shifts.

The person in charge, either the sister or staff nurse, made sure that we never missed a meal, something that today's staff simply accept. We were never allowed to eat on the wards, but the ward sisters were usually as generous as they could be in giving us breaks. If we weren't too busy, we were encouraged to go to the canteen for a morning coffee and more often for tea halfway through an afternoon shift, as well as once at night.

The dining room was on the ground floor of the nurses' home, where we'd collect our meal at a serving hatch. There wasn't a choice like in a canteen. We got what we were given, though a different meal with a pudding was served every day. They were good meals and they were free, so we couldn't complain. Everyone looked forward to going to the dining room and wanted to know what was on the menu from the people who'd already been that day.

The sisters and Matron ate in a separate room. Although there were no obvious divisions in the rest of the large room, there was an unwritten rule that the most junior nurses sat furthest from the serving area and the staff nurses and senior nurses used the tables nearest it. Generally we'd look for a member of our set or someone we'd worked with so that we could sit and eat with them.

On one of my weekend days off, I had a treat as Jackie Stone came to visit me. It had been seven years since I had seen her last at primary school. Jackie remembers us having lunch in the nurses' dining room. I recall that when the staff on duty had finished coming for their meals, off-duty staff could have a meal there and even bring a friend. No food was wasted.

Jackie remembers me eating my food very quickly. I apparently told her that we were not always allocated much time for our meal breaks. Jackie and I then spent some time in my room in the nurses' home, chatting, catching up and enjoying each other's company. Jackie was working for one of Lloyd's insurance brokers in London, recording data. She had become engaged to her boyfriend, Ken, two years before in 1961, aged 17. They are still married today. Apparently I told Jackie about how we practised giving injections into oranges and she exclaimed, "A poor orange that couldn't fight back!" It was a lovely day but went far too quickly.

Throughout our practical training, we always carried our booklet of competencies – *Record of Practical Instruction for the Certificate of Nursing Sick Children* – produced by the General Nursing Council for England and Wales, our registration body. We referred to this booklet as our "cross-chart". It contained 153 printed competencies, which were signed off by the ward sisters or the sister tutors. Once one of these competencies was taught in class, it had to be marked in the cross-chart. Afterwards we were shown the procedure on the ward and a line and initial was added. Finally, the line was crossed and initialled when we were deemed competent at the procedure.

The competencies ranged from feeding children in the first year to the application of skin and skeletal traction (a way of treating broken bones) and the administration of medicines in the final year. As we finished on a ward, the sister made sure our charts were up to date and the competencies we had achieved were signed. There was a section in the back for her to write details of any "special experiences".

We had a sister tutor who worked regularly with us. All the sister tutors wore uniform as they were teaching us procedures and testing our knowledge on the wards themselves. They were very up to date with everything that went on. This helped us because Matron would regularly take a student on a ward round, making sure she knew all about her patients, including all their test results. This was especially frequent and nerve-racking on night duty when she had more time to spend with a student.

My experience with the thermometer kept me on my toes. I would be asked to take Matron on a ward round, accompanying her from patient to patient, telling her the name, age and diagnoses of all 20 children on the ward and giving an up-to-date report on each child's condition and treatment. We weren't allowed to refer to our ward handover notebook; everything had to be done from memory. I remember doing this a number of times, but always on night duty.

Matron would get an update of the patients at the end of the day from the ward sister (or a staff nurse if the sister was off duty). This would then be passed on to the night sisters. That way she'd have an understanding of how well we students knew our patients and whether we were up to date with their progress. There was no escape, nowhere to hide.

Every child admitted to the hospital had to have their hair examined for nits, which were rife in London children at that time and spread like mad. The surgeons and anaesthetists were repulsed by head lice, terrified of catching them while leaning over a child in the theatre. They most certainly did *not* want to take them home so we, the nurses, had to make sure that infected children were treated before they were allowed on the operating table.

We could often spot the telltale sign of the eggs, but not usually the lice. Even so, we wet each child's hair and combed it through with a special fine-tooth comb, quickly trying to capture anything we found in a tissue. We had to be thorough.

On another ward at the time, an anaesthetist actually sent a child back from theatre when he spotted nits in her hair. There was no way he would consider sitting close to her head until she'd been treated. Even though we did this persistent, contagious procedure regularly, "competent at identifying and treating nits" was never written in my competency book under special experiences!

While the making of beds and the sterilising of bottles and potties was our early-morning chore, the rest of the day was spent keeping up with the routine observations on the children and learning the specialist care of the children admitted to the ward for surgery. There were patients I remember observing on 4C&D which, unknown to me then, would have a special place in my future nursing career.

LEARNING ON THE JOB

On the ward, we nursed babies born with a cleft lip and palate, a gap in their lip and the roof of their mouth. A child would be returned to the ward following a repair to a cleft lip with a bow of metal across their lip to take the tension off the wound. If the child was being breastfed, the metal bow had to be loosened before feeds. Otherwise the child was spoon-fed. Their lip had to be cleaned regularly, especially after feeds.

For the first 24 hours, the child would also have a stitch through the centre of their tongue, the ends of which were stuck with plaster to their cheek. This was especially done following the palate repair in case there were problems with the child's airway. Their tongue could then be pulled forward using the stitch. Although I was involved in their care, I was never allowed to be left on my own with these children as they needed more experienced staff to look after them, especially with feeding.

The cleft lip and palate children were referred to Mr Matthews, our consultant plastic surgeon. He was renowned for his excellent surgery. Many other babies with congenital problems throughout Britain were referred to him, particularly those needing facial reconstruction. When Mr Matthews retired, Mr Broomhead, his registrar while we were training, took over Mr Matthew's good work and continued GOS's reputation.

I was given the opportunity to look after some of the children admitted for plastic surgery. These were the children who'd had surgery to separate fused fingers, remove large moles and various swellings, and pin back ears. Another common operation was plastic surgery to scars following burns, particularly those causing a tightening of the skin that reduced how well an arm or a hand worked.

There were also children on 4C&D who'd undergone eye surgery. What I remember was the correction of squints. Children would come in looking very cross-eyed, and even though their eyes were red after their surgery, they returned home looking and feeling infinitely better. I felt very satisfied to see the results of all the cosmetic surgery. School can be a cruel-enough place for children.

There was one particular newborn baby with a much rarer condition. When she was admitted, she was placed in a side room with the curtains drawn. There was an atmosphere of apprehension on the ward. We students couldn't understand what was going on. Eventually, each student was taken to see this baby. She had been born with an abnormally formed forebrain. It was the most severe form, and she was what was known as a Cyclops.

I was heartbroken at the sight of this newborn with only one eye in the centre of her forehead, and I couldn't stop thinking about her parents who had to make such a horrendous choice. At that time at GOS, a decision would have been made in conjunction with the parents to allow the child to die as quickly and as peacefully as possible. Today, any child with this condition would be diagnosed at the first prenatal ultrasound scan of the pregnancy and a termination would be offered on medical grounds.

Seeing this child, though, helped me in later life. My husband was a parish priest in Bermondsey, southeast London. Men who lived on the streets regularly came to our building. One day, when I was alone, there was a knock on the front door. I peeped through the spy hole to see who it was. I was amazed to see a grown man who was a Cyclops. I partially opened the door, keeping the chain on, and asked if I could help him.

"Please could I have something to eat and drink?" He was polite and non-threatening. So once I'd established whether he wanted tea or coffee and what he'd like in his sandwich, I opened the door to give him a chair in our enclosed porch.

"Have a seat while I make you that sandwich," I said.

He sat down and looked comfortable enough but, when I returned with the tray, the chair was empty. He'd gone.

I opened the front door to see if he was perhaps waiting outside and I spotted him walking down the road. Without thinking, I left the tray and ran after him.

"Hello," I said once I'd caught up with him. "I've made your sandwich."

"Oh," he said. "I'd forgotten about that."

Remembering that little baby, I wanted to do something for him, however small a gesture. "Come back with me?" I suggested. "It's cheese and pickle, just like you asked."

He said he'd be glad to and we walked back together towards our home.

In those days, we had community police who knew us well. They stopped in a Panda car and wound down the window.

"You all right, Mrs Martin?" the driver asked.

I went over to them. "Yes, I'm fine, thank you. I'm just giving this gentleman tea and a sandwich."

They looked at him, then back at me, assessing the situation. "We'll circle the block to keep an eye on you," one of them said.

It was considerate and reassuring of them, but I had no fear of this man. He was softly spoken with a mild manner. How on earth did he survive on the streets? What had brought him to this point?

I never found out. We never saw him again. But this was a long time in the future. Marriage and the birth of two boys was going to intervene.

While I was on 4C&D, my dentist had been concerned because one of my second teeth had grown through my palate behind a front baby tooth that I had never lost. He knew I was working at GOS and referred me to their orthodontic department, which was in the outpatients department. This department was one of very few units who, at that time, were experimenting in moving children's misaligned teeth to improve their smile.

My dentist asked the orthodontists whether it would be worth them moving this tooth in my palate rather than taking it out, as it was in a very awkward place. The senior orthodontist at GOS warned me that this would be experimental, but he would like to try it. If it worked, he told me, with my own tooth in that position, it should last me a lifetime. I agreed to let them take my baby tooth out and move the tooth in my palate.

I was fitted for a plate to wear in my mouth; it had a

movable part that could be turned with a key. Once a week, I had to visit the department so that they could turn the key to put pressure on my tooth and gradually move it into the correct position. My mouth and the appliance were photographed every month.

My mouth became quite famous. I would sometimes be phoned on 4C&D and Sister O'Mara would be asked if she could spare me to be examined by a visiting orthodontist. It took six months to move my tooth and six months of my having to talk with a lisp! The department got to know me well. Today, no one would know that the tooth hadn't grown in its place originally.

I was still on 4C&D when Christmas came. Preparations at GOS began in mid-December. Staff volunteered to paint the cubicle windows on the ward and they would come in on their own time to do this. It was clear who the artists were when amazing Disney scenes appeared, brightening up all the wards. The hospital itself had a group that organised a nativity play. They would usually find a few children who were well enough to take part in it, which always made it really special.

The doctors always put on a revue in the dining hall in the nurses' home. They wrote sketches based on different situations in the hospital and mimicked consultants whom they felt were tolerant enough to laugh with all of us. This show was always popular and well attended. Off-duty nurses volunteered to do a procession of carol singing around the wards on Christmas Eve. They wore their uniforms with their capes inside out, showing the festive red. I was even able to teach my new friends and colleagues some carols in German. They got quite good at "Stille Nacht".

4C&D's theme that year was Snow White and the Seven Dwarfs. Staff made their own costumes and dressed up to accompany Father Christmas around the wards. They would begin on Christmas morning, walking up the hospital drive with Father Christmas, and we would take all the children who were well enough onto the balcony to wave at him.

The decorations and the tree on Christmas Day were spectacular. We staff were expected to work all Christmas Day and Boxing Day. No leave was allowed. A cosy corner was erected, usually in the corner of one of the wards, where we could sit and eat on these two days as the canteen was shut.

It was tradition on Christmas Day for the senior consultant of each ward to come to the hospital with his family. When the turkey came up from the kitchen, he would wear a decorated hat while carving it, and then he would serve the turkey to all the children, parents and staff. I discovered later that on some wards it was tradition to invite a patient or two who were regulars (and either had a disability or were poor) to come with their families and join in with the Christmas meal.

Meanwhile, around all these celebrations, the BBC were setting up their live outside broadcasting equipment. Their vans were in the drive to the entrance of the hospital and technicians were laying cables that were being manoeuvred up ladders and through windows. This was a regular Christmas Day programme in the 1960s called *Meeting the Kids in Hospital this Christmas* and was screened at 2 p.m. before the Queen's Speech.

Max Bygraves gave out presents to the children in the hospital. He was very popular with the staff and children

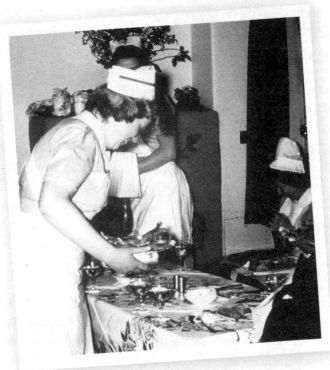

Serving up Christmas dinner.

alike and could always persuade the patients to talk to him. It was the role of a staff member on each ward to find a child who was well and articulate enough to be presented to Max and be given an amazing present, which would come from the store of donations given to the hospital. Max would also attend a ward or two with a cameraman if there was a cute or very articulate child who was bed bound.

Christmas was over very quickly. By the end of New Year's Day, all decorations were down and the windows spotlessly clean. It was back to normal.

My three-month period on Ward 4C&D was over and the time came for me to move to my second ward. Moving wards was always a scary time for us. I'd gradually built up relationships with the staff on 4C&D and the ward was familiar to me. It was now time to move on and learn new skills.

My second ward was on the ground floor. Cohen Ward took the patients with infections and had a number of cubicles in which children were isolated. Here I learnt the strict rules of infection control. In the School of Nursing, we had learnt the technique of good handwashing, wearing a mask and putting on a gown, to protect all the babies under six months from infection. On Cohen, we were taught strict barrier nursing for any child who had an infection.

In their cubicle, each child had their own crockery onto which food and drink were transferred, their own cutlery and their own medicine pots into which the medicine was measured. All waste was double-bagged and, when children were discharged, their toys had to be tragically thrown away. We had to warn parents about this and try to find a way of preserving special toys as this could be quite upsetting for a child.

Looking back, I can see how all the infection control procedures saved lives. I can't help but wonder if we could have beaten coronavirus more quickly if everyone had been trained as we were.

There are two ways of preventing the spread of infection. One way is barrier nursing, which we practised on Cohen Ward. This prevents a patient's infection from spreading to us and other patients on the ward. The other way was then known as reverse barrier nursing, which was used to prevent a child in isolation from getting an infection from outside.

Reverse barrier nursing was used on all babies under six months who were nursed in cubicles at GOS. Both of these involved the same techniques that we were taught in preliminary training school and then tested on later in our training blocks and on the wards.

We all have to get used to wearing masks these days. In the 1960s, in the hospitals I worked in, masks were kept in dispensers outside the cubicles. We would take and put on the mask using the ties without touching and contaminating the mask itself. We opened the swing door to the cubicle by pushing it with an elbow or going in backwards. Next, we would handwash for a minimum of 30 seconds (two 'Happy Birthdays'!), also something that is becoming second nature to us all.

We wore no jewellery. The only ring allowed was a single band (for married women when GOS eventually employed them), which had to be washed carefully underneath. And no wristwatches – only a fob watch pinned to our uniform. Nails had to be very short so that they couldn't be seen at all if we looked at our hands with the palms facing us and absolutely no nail polish was allowed.

One day in our training school, the microbiology department sent a microbiologist to test how well we washed our hands. He used swabs to take samples from between our fingers and thumbs and under our nails to see if he could grow any bacteria from our hands. I don't think he managed to, which was a relief to us all, so our handwashing must have been efficiently performed. He did show us samples of bacteria he had grown from unwashed hands, which brought home to us just how much we carried on unclean hands.

After masks and hands, we had to put on a gown. This hung on a hanger on a coat hook on the wall behind the door. It had an open back and hung with the back towards us. To put on the gown, we slipped our arms through the sleeves without touching anything but the inside of the gown. The gown covered the whole of our uniform and we did it up at the back (like a gown a patient wears to go to theatre now).

If another ward in the hospital had an infection or had another reason for a good clean, we students occasionally helped. I remember once having to spend a day scrubbing everything until it was spotless. The ward cleaners took down the curtains to be sent to the hospital laundry and scrubbed all the skirting boards, walls and floors in the empty ward.

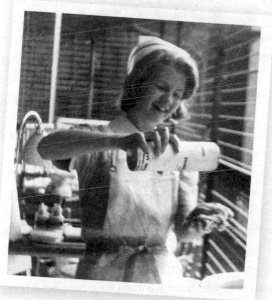

Me with the scouring powder.

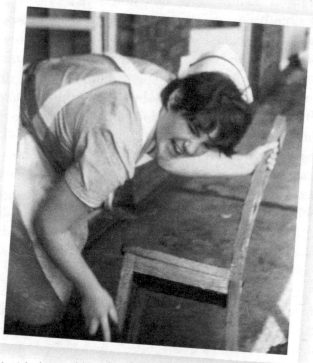

Carol with the scrubbing brush.

Although it was gruelling work, we quite enjoyed the rare chance to let our hair down and have a laugh.

Cohen Ward had a baby who was being nursed in an incubator while I was there. Though I have a picture of her, I remember little about her. But I do remember an 18-month-old boy with red hair – at that time, he was the youngest child ever to have been diagnosed with type 1 diabetes. Everyone loved him as he smiled all the time and had a lovely nature. It was hard for him to have regular injections of insulin at that age, but he coped incredibly well.

We also had children with bowel problems. I learnt how to feel, very gently, for impacted faeces (poo stuck in the bowel) and how to give glycerine suppositories to help them on their way. We used finger cots instead of the disposable plastic gloves used today. Finger cots were like a small condom, which we would roll down over the middle finger of our right hand for the procedure. I also learnt how to perform an enema, a washout that involved putting a rubber tube into a child's backside, then pouring a measured amount of warm water into the bowel through a funnel. We would then immediately reverse the tube and funnel so that the water and the faeces could be evacuated into a bucket.

I also had my first experience of checking medicines on the medicine round. This was a much longer procedure on an infectious ward. I would have to check the medicine with the staff nurse, and she would have to walk with me to the cubicle door of the child who was isolating. She would check with me that I had the right patient before I gave the child the medicine. I would put on my mask, transfer the medicine into the medicine pot in the child's cubicle before going through the procedure of handwashing and gowning up and giving the child the medicine.

I had learnt a great deal on Cohen Ward about different bacteria and viruses and how they were spread. I learnt how to protect yourself and others from them and the very serious complications that could result from catching them. I was lucky enough not to experience the death of a child on that ward, but deaths from serious infections were not uncommon in the hospital.

NIGHT DUTY

After three months on Cohen Ward, our next three months were to be spent on night duty. Another new ward experience, where we could meet new people and learn new skills. This time we had to adjust our body clocks to sleeping during the day and working 12-hour shifts at night for eight nights in a row. Luckily the nurses' home was well insulated and quiet during the day, and this enabled us to sleep well.

I wasn't particularly looking forward to this three-month stretch of nights as I'd heard how tiring it was. But it had to be done every year. My turn had arrived. I was to spend it on 2ABE, a medical ward. Because each ward had two sides to it, each with six children and four babies, a third-year student would take charge of the ward and was responsible for the busiest side. A second-year student would take responsibility for the other side – their first introduction to management. The first-year student would run between the two sides and do whatever she was asked. This was to be my role.

The previous first-year student always left a list in your pigeonhole of all the patients who had been on the ward the night before. It would include their names, ages, diagnoses, on-going treatment and test results. This was my first experience of night duty. I found that the first-year student from the set above me, who was just finishing her three-month stretch of nights, had left a very comprehensive written handover report of all the children on 2ABE in my pigeonhole. I never met this student and didn't know who she was, but I was very grateful for the trouble that she took.

I tried to memorise all the names of the children and as much as I could about them before that night shift, to prepare myself for this new experience. It was essential to learn all this off by heart. Not only did the night sisters want to know that you knew all the patients, but of course we knew that Matron would do a round once a night and choose a nurse on one of the wards to test. You were reprimanded if you did not have this information at your fingertips.

The third-year student in charge of 2ABE was particularly welcoming and helpful. She took real concern over my health. She made sure that both the second-year student and I took our breaks and had plenty to drink during our night shifts. She was also concerned about our sleep; as she lived in one of the outside residential homes, I think her accommodation was noisier than ours. After one of my night shifts, she was telling me that I was far too pale and I should get some sunshine to top up my vitamin D levels. She insisted that I should go up on to the roof of the nurses' home and spend some time in the sun.

"I want to see more colour in your cheeks tonight when you come back on duty," she told me. I only did it once as I have fair skin which began to burn.

There was a much quieter atmosphere on the wards at night, except for the lift, which had old-fashioned metal doors and rattled as it moved from floor to floor. The sound of the lift starting up and moving through the shaft alerted us to the possibility of one of the sisters or Matron doing ward rounds or perhaps an emergency admission. Staff didn't miss what was happening at night in their block, that's for sure. As students, we were encouraged to use the stairs, so usually we only used the lift to take a child to the operating theatres on the sixth floor.

There were about 17 wards over seven floors in the hospital. Four night sisters had overall responsibility for the care of all the children on these wards. It was compulsory in those days for anyone wanting to become a ward sister and have overall 24-hour responsibility of a ward, its staff, the junior doctors and the patients, to have been a night sister for at least a year before applying for this senior post. The night sisters would do a regular round, checking the medicines with us on their allocated wards and helping out if they were needed. In later years they carried a bleep for us to call them, but in my training days we would phone the switchboard, which then set two numbers on all the clocks in the hospital to flash intermittently to call our night sister.

These clocks were unique to GOS, which was the only hospital to have developed a "call system". They could be used to call a team to a child who had had a respiratory arrest (they stopped breathing) or cardiac arrest (their heart stopped beating). Clocks were situated in every corridor and ward of the hospital. The night sisters and doctors would know which numbers were theirs and could respond immediately to the flashing numbers.

One morning, at the end of eight nights of night duty when we were due to have our time off, Julia asked me if I'd go with her to Matins in the hospital chapel.

"I'd love to," I said.

St Christopher's was (and still is) a spectacular and highly decorated Victorian chapel. We'd visited it before, but never attended a service there. Such a beautiful and calm space for the children, with its child-sized pews and collection of soft toys to hold the children's attention. The peaceful, gold interior was a sanctuary for weary and sometimes distressed families and staff.

As soon as I walked into the chapel, I felt how calm it was, but not for long. I realised that I'd forgotten to bring any collection. We weren't in the habit of carrying money and, although Julia had a coin with her, she had nothing extra she could lend me. It was a nice service and I'd relaxed, but then: "Oh, no. Please, no."

During the last hymn, I spotted Matron. She was taking the collection. Why was she always present at my most embarrassing moments? Luckily she was passing round a bag and not a plate. I put my hand into the bag and pretended to give an offering, but I knew that the colour in my cheeks was giving me away. Matron behaved impeccably.

2ABE mainly treated children with cancer. I remember very clearly a baby boy with leukaemia whom I nursed for a few weeks. He was such a bonny boy with a lovely temperament. Luckily, most children with this type of leukaemia are cured today,[7] but there was no known cure for it at that time.

The book that we had to buy to use in the nursing school explained that new medicines were constantly being tried, but the results were disappointing. The medicine cortisone would "temporarily arrest the course of the disease, but because the case was hopeless the nurse must not relax her efforts to keep the child comfortable".[11] Because there was no cure for leukaemia, medical institutions deliberately withheld information from the public about this serious illness.[7]

It wasn't until 1960 that the first stories of children fighting cancer started to feature in the national press. Following the loss of their daughter to what was then known as acute leukaemia, two remarkable parents founded a charity, the Teesside Leukaemia Fund. With the first £5,000 they funded the opening of a leukaemia research unit in December 1961 at the Hospital for Sick Children in Great Ormond Street. The stories about this new charity unleashed a flood of public inquiries from relatives of children with the disease and from members of the public wishing to raise funds.[7]

Sadly, one night when I was on duty, the baby boy I had been nursing died. I'd got to know him well over the last few weeks and, although it was clear he wouldn't survive this awful disease, it was still a shock. This was the first death I had experienced and I was determined to be as calm and professional as I could be.

We laid him out. It was difficult, but I put my feelings to one side and concentrated on the job at hand. I was determined to do my best for him, the last thing I could do, with Great Ormond Street attention to detail. Performing the last offices (care given to the body after death) helps with coming to terms with the death of a child, because you are doing something practical for both the child and the parents. There is something almost ritualistic about carrying out procedures such as these, giving some sense of order to what is often the worst of situations. When we are involved in tragedies we cannot change, scrupulous care and procedures can bring some comfort.

The first thing we did was to close a child's eyes with damp cotton wool balls and, if the mouth was open, bandage the jaw closed. The cotton wool and bandage would be left in place until rigor mortis set in because only then will the eyes and mouth remain closed. Meanwhile, we washed and dried the child's body, making sure that any wounds were redressed, etc. We would then dress the child in a hospital shroud or, if the parents had particular clothes that they wished the child to be dressed in, we'd use those. We brushed the child's hair and for a girl, if requested, put the hair into bunches or plaits. Then we'd fold the arms across the chest and place the hands in a praying position with fingers together.

Downstairs in the hospital foyer, there was always a display of white flowers in a vase, for the use of staff in such a situation. The parents were given a time to come to the hospital to see their child. Just before they came, we would collect a flower to put in the child's hands. If the child was a girl, we might take a second flower to put in her hair. It was amazing how beautiful the children looked, and the parents often remarked on this.

The night the baby died, after we'd placed one of the white flowers in his clasped hands, I went into the sluice. I let myself give in to those bottled-up emotions and cried.

"Nurse Owen, what do you think you are doing? Pull yourself together."

It was the night sister.

"You must learn to hold in your feelings," she said, firmly but not unkindly. "One day it will be your duty to support the family and other staff through this experience."

"I'm sorry, Sister."

"Now wash your face and return to your duties."

And with that I was left alone in the sluice. How many other nurses had sought refuge in here in the same situation? Had Sister or Matron ever felt like this?

I always remembered those remarks, always remembered this duty, but it never stopped me from being upset after the death of a child.

I'd been working on 2ABE for about four weeks when an eight-year-old boy, Jeremy, was admitted as an emergency to the ward. He'd fallen in the garden onto a sycamore tree stump, cutting his lip and gums and filling his mouth with soil. Ten days later, his GP referred him as an emergency to GOS with swelling around his eyes and slurred speech. The GP had realised the seriousness of Jeremy's symptoms.

Jeremy was seen by a senior registrar, who reported that the boy had difficulty opening his mouth and swallowing. He had the facial appearance of tetanus (often referred to as lockjaw) with a swollen mouth and cheeks, half-closed eyes and slow facial movements. Tetanus is a serious infection, caused by bacteria found in soil. The toxins from the bacteria affect the tissues of the nervous system, causing swelling around the face and neck and spasms, particularly of the throat and neck muscles, which can lead to severe breathing problems. Tetanus can be fatal if it is not treated quickly. In the early 1960s, children frequently died of the infection.

I asked the ward sister if I could use Jeremy as my first-year patient study. It was agreed that I could, so I was allowed to be present for most of his care at night and to assist the staff nurse who was "specialling" him. All very sick children were "specialled". This meant they were given one-to-one care in a side room of a ward by a registered sick children's trained nurse.

Jeremy was admitted to 2E, an extension to the main ward with six cubicles. He had the ward to himself. Noise, bright lights and anything that would startle him could cause him to have painful muscle spasms, so the ward was adapted especially for him.

"Quiet Please" notices were hung up outside the doors, and other children were kept away from the area. The telephone ring was dulled. We lowered our voices at all times. We weren't allowed to wear noisy shoes. Jeremy's cubicle was darkened by hanging large red blankets in front of each window and the lighting inside the ward was dimmed.

All of this was intended to help control some of Jeremy's muscle spasms. Spasms in his jaw wouldn't only cause breathing problems, but also made swallowing difficult and caused him to bite his tongue. Spasms in his back muscles would cause him to arch his back and cry out in pain. Everything had to be as calm and as quiet as it could possibly be. Jeremy's sister was told by her mother that a doctor slept outside Jeremy's room on a camp bed. I remember one of the on-call registrars using the next-door cubicle as his on-call rest room for the first few nights so that he could be available for Jeremy if he was needed.

Jeremy received four different medicines. He was given an antibiotic, intramuscular penicillin, four times a day. I sympathised with him as I too had to have this injection in my backside when I was in the staff sick bay. Tetanus antitoxin was given into a vein; this helped Jeremy's body to produce antibodies to fight the bacteria, just as our vaccines for Covid help us to produce antibodies against the virus today. He received medicine to prevent him vomiting as this could stop him breathing. Finally, he had a sedative medicine that had a calming effect to help control his muscle spasms.

Jeremy began by having his calming medicine in suppository form (into his bottom). This was not pleasant for him so the medical staff changed it to a liquid form that he could swallow. I witnessed his first dose as it was given at 10 p.m. at night. It must have tasted extremely nasty because, immediately after taking it, Jeremy had a five-minute spasm that made him go completely rigid. He shouted so loudly that the night sisters could hear him downstairs in their office. The medicine was immediately changed back into suppository form.

Jeremy had these spasms for four of the five weeks that he was in hospital. Normally, before a spasm, he would cry out, his jaw would become tight and set and he would screw up his face and bite his tongue. Then he'd fling his body around and clench his fists, crying out at the same time. These spasms usually lasted from about 10 seconds to a few minutes. We had to time each spasm and record on a chart how it affected him.

He needed a great deal of reassurance, especially as his parents, twin brother and sister were unable to visit as often as they would have liked. He'd cry bitterly following a spasm, partly from the pain, as often his tongue was so badly bitten it was bleeding, but also from sheer exhaustion. Jeremy can still remember to this day the spasms and biting the end of his tongue badly.

Jeremy had to survive on special milk, which was sent up from the diet kitchen. He managed to drink this along with tepid water (though he says he preferred Ribena to the water) through a straw. Because his face was so swollen, we could only just manage to push the straw into one corner of his mouth. This was his food for three long weeks. After that he was able to eat soft food from the ward food trolley keep.

Jeremy was on Ward 2ABE for five of my 12 weeks on night duty. For two of these weeks, he was specialled. When he could manage without his trained nurse specialling him, he was overseen by a third-year student. I was able to continue performing much of his routine care while still carrying out my normal duties on both sides of the ward with the remaining children.

Gradually, the numbers of Jeremy's spasms were decreasing. During the fifth week they became much less frequent, most of them occurring at night, until there were eventually none at all. We would then find him sitting up in the main ward when we came on duty. We were witnessing him becoming quite cheeky and playing pranks, which showed he was recovering.

Jeremy wrote to me recently. He said, "Of course I have no recollection of any cheekiness at all!"

Parents in those days only visited their children for an hour each evening, but they could come at other times at the discretion of the ward sister or when they asked (or were invited) to speak to the medical staff. I did meet Jeremy's parents but not his siblings. If parents were present while we were nursing their child, especially if they were very ill, we had lots of interaction with them. But mostly we would only talk to parents at visiting time. This way they felt they had some control over the care of their child without a member of staff breathing down their necks, and they could spend quality time with their child.

When Jeremy's family visited, they brought him a number of games to play. His older sister wrote him letters regularly, informing him of everything she'd been doing and the things he'd missed at home. She even brought him up to date with the flowers and plants that had come up in his own patch of garden. During his time in hospital, Jeremy also had one of the hospital schoolteachers visiting him regularly. Maths was a favourite subject of his, and we would often find him doing his maths homework when we came on duty.

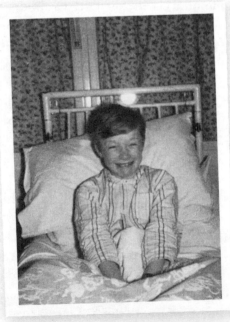

Jeremy five days before being discharged home. He still has swelling around his eyes.

When Jeremy was discharged home, he remembers that it wasn't winter anymore and the trees had leaves on them. After he was discharged, I wrote to his mother, asking for a photo of him to include in my study. She wrote back, sending me a photo and saying how much she owed to the hospital and how grateful she was for the love and care given to her son. She remarked that he'd not only recovered physically, but had emerged from hospital a more independent, outgoing boy. Jeremy provided me with a subject for an interesting patient-care study and I even acquired a highly sought-after A for my work.

This was 1963. The tetanus vaccine was only introduced routinely in 1961 and even then not to children of Jeremy's age. Today it's given as part of a combination vaccine in a

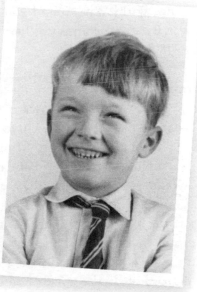

Jeremy aged six and a half, given to me by his mother.

routine immunisation programme for children, starting at the age of two months. Although tetanus is a notifiable disease, cases are known to be under-reported. Nevertheless, from January to December 2018, only seven cases were reported in England. All were adults aged between 31 and 88 years of age. Of the seven cases, six were born before 1961 and the other case was an intravenous drug user. Three cases died from their infection.[8]

Technology was also far less advanced in 1963; there were no intensive care units. Today we have paediatric intensive care units (PICUs) in children's hospitals. Here, medical staff will have the use of medicines that paralyse the muscles to prevent spasms, and a ventilator to breathe for the child if these medicines are used. These developments have helped to prevent the death of patients with tetanus. Before the Second World War, around 200 people died of tetanus each year. By 1970, tetanus was hardly seen at all in children in the UK.[9]

My three-months night duty was coming to an end and I was ready for a break. We were to have a two-week holiday and I'd arranged to go back to Geesthacht to visit the family I had worked for as an au pair. Before I finished my night duty, I asked the night sister for the name of the first-year student who would replace me on the ward. She would be from the January 1963 set, one below me. I wrote a handover report for her on the children with their names, ages, diagnoses and anything else I knew about them, just as the student in the set above me had done for me. I left the report in her pigeonhole in the nurses' home.

After a good sleep following those last eight nights of the shift, I travelled on the night ferry from Harwich to Hook in Holland, sharing a cabin with a German girl. We were chatting in German when a steward came to tell us that he would wake us at five o'clock in the morning, so we'd be ready to leave the boat when we docked in Hook.

"Gosh, that's early to have to get up," I said.

"Your English is very good," he replied.

I was really rather pleased that he'd thought I was German, but, when I told this tale to the Beckers, they laughed uncontrollably, particularly Christian. They even recounted this incident to all their friends. I was surprised at their hilarity as I only thought it mildly amusing. Presumably the steward thought my German was good enough for me to pass as a native, though because I was fair-haired, it wasn't the only time this mistake took place.

It was lovely to see the family. The youngest, Dinah, was now three years old and had grown so much. The other two were well established at school and trying out their English on me. The family took me sightseeing; we spent a day in Lübeck and visited the large cathedral there, which was very impressive. It had been partly destroyed during the Second World War and their impressive organ was destroyed by fire. The cathedral had been reconstructed and the organ rebuilt. I would have liked to have heard the organ being played but didn't get that opportunity.

It was a lovely break and I had been looked after so well, enjoying many of Frau Becker's amazing cakes. The return journey was uneventful (no stewards to impress) and the ferry crossing home was a smooth one.

I returned to GOS to spend three months on the last ward of my first year, 7C&D, the ear, nose and throat (ENT) ward. This ward had its own theatre attached to it and I knew that I would have some theatre experience while looking after patients. I'd been warned to have a good breakfast every morning as the surgeon did not take kindly to staff who fainted in his theatre. Many children were admitted for the removal of their tonsils and adenoids, which were commonly removed together at that time. I was able to do the admission of a child, take him to theatre, watch the operation and recover him before taking him back to the ward to look after him.

I remember the children having tongue clips in place while we recovered them so that their tongue could be pulled forward if they had breathing difficulties. Tongue clips were rather barbaric instruments with two sharp clips on scissor handles. They were clipped to the centre of the tongue and could only be removed when the child objected to them, which they always did as soon as they were awake enough to feel them.

It was good to follow children right through their care, from admission to discharge. In theatre, the children were anaesthetised by inhaling ether. A mask was placed over their nose and mouth with gauze covering it and ether was then slowly dripped onto the mask until the child became unconscious. Then their tonsils and adenoids were quickly removed.

It was a very speedy process with four to six children being operated on in one theatre session. The problem was the ether. Its smell lingered on the patient's breath and in the ward for hours afterwards. But worse than this were the fumes, which dizzyingly filled the theatre. Mr James Crooks, our consultant ENT surgeon, did *not* like any noise in the theatre. If anyone looked as though they might possibly faint, they were quickly and quietly removed before they tumbled to the floor with a crash.

It was on this ward that I learnt to nurse children with a tracheostomy, an artificial opening into the windpipe. With the staff nurse, I learnt how to suction the tracheostomy tube carefully and safely using an aseptic technique, how to care for the stoma (the opening into the windpipe) and how to change the tapes holding the tracheostomy in place.

I nursed a baby with a tracheostomy. She'd originally been admitted with noisy breathing, known as a "stridor". On examination in theatre, she was found to have a cyst in her windpipe – this was causing the stridor. The cyst was removed. The baby was given a temporary tracheostomy until the area had healed and the surgeon was sure she'd have no further breathing problems. While helping to care for this baby, I perfected my technique of reverse barrier nursing (protecting the patient from infection) that I'd previously learnt.

I had two other very interesting learning experiences on this ward, both emergency admissions. The first was a young boy of about four years with an abscess in the area behind his throat. This unusual infection can come on very quickly. An abscess found here can lead to severe breathing problems and even result in death. He was rushed to theatre by the consultant surgeon to have his abscess incised (cut) and drained without causing further complications – a technique that requires both skill and precision. He was returned from theatre to the ward on oxygen with an intravenous infusion and on antibiotics. He was specialled for the night but recovered within a few days with no lasting effects.

The second emergency was a newborn baby admitted with severe breathing problems and unable to feed. She was diagnosed with choanal atresia, a rare condition in which the nasal passages haven't developed properly and are blocked with either tissue or bone. Babies use their nose for breathing and use their mouth to attach to the breast to suckle efficiently. For this reason babies under six months have to be able to breathe through their nose and cannot mouth breathe effectively.[10] This baby had to have an airway (a plastic breathing tube) fixed into her mouth so she could breathe. She also needed a feeding tube put through her mouth and into her stomach. These artificial methods of breathing and feeding were continued while the surgeon arranged investigations as to why she had this severe nasal blockage. It also allowed time for the baby to gain weight and be fit enough to cope with an operation. An examination and X-ray discovered both of her nostrils were blocked with bone.

When the baby had gained enough weight, I was allowed to accompany her to theatre to watch the operation. The noise-hating Mr Crooks drilled through the offending bone to open up her nostrils. I remember feeling quite queasy at the sound of the drill going through the bone but knew I couldn't move a muscle. I certainly couldn't risk fainting. Once the drilling was completed, I could focus once more on the operation and watch the plastic tubes being inserted and then stitched into both nostrils. This would keep the nasal passages open and allow the baby to breathe on her own. Despite his eccentricity, I couldn't help but admire Mr Crooks's skill.

Over the next few weeks, this baby gradually learnt to feed and enjoy it. The nursing staff regularly used suction to remove any fluid from the plastic tubes to keep them open. Once the tubes were removed and the area operated on had healed and once the baby was feeding well and gaining weight, she was discharged home.

At the end of 12 weeks, I had finished my experience on 7C&D. All too soon, our first year of training was over. We were straight into our second year and back in the nursing school for our six-week block of teaching.

SECOND YEAR

Before the teaching began, the tutors checked our cross-charts to make sure we had achieved our first-year competencies and signed them off. The rest of our teaching in the nursing school was based on a comprehensive Great Ormond Street book that we all had to have bought called *Nursing and Diseases of Sick Children*.[11] It was written with the help of GOS medical and nursing staff, the latter of which, as the editors admitted, were not included in the list of contributors.

Our introductory preliminary training school lectures had given us the basic knowledge we needed to begin our work on the wards. Teaching from now on would be more geared to the specific diseases of children. We would have the consultant physicians and surgeons who had written the chapters in the book lecturing to us. They were specialists in the field, so the lectures were in great depth. We would meet the consultants over the coming year. They treated us as they would have done junior doctors, so we had to keep alert.

Burns and plastic surgery was taught by Mr David Matthews, who had invited me to join him on his ward round. Mr James Crooks (who couldn't abide noise in his theatre) lectured us on diseases of the ear, nose and throat.

Common medical diseases, particularly of the newborn, were taught by Professor Alan Moncrieff, orthopaedic surgery by Mr George Lloyd-Roberts and urinary diseases by Mr David Innes Williams, the last three of whom I had yet to meet on their wards. I also remember being lectured by a senior consultant anaesthetist called Miss Margaret Hawksley, who was head of the anaesthetic department. It was unusual to have a woman in such a high position in those days.

One consultant who sticks out in my mind was renowned child psychologist, Dr Mildred Creak. She was given the first post as physician in psychological medicine at GOS in 1946. She must have taught us in our block just before she retired as I remember that she was the first person to introduce us to the condition of autism. At the time, autism was called "schizophrenic syndrome of childhood", a mental condition thought to be caused by parental inadequacy, a professional belief that caused considerable suffering to parents. Before her retirement, Dr Creak had studied 100 children diagnosed with autism, concluding that the condition was *not* a mental one but was primarily due to genetic coding present at birth. This has since been confirmed by scientific evidence.[12] The Mildred Creak Unit was built in memory of her work and is the hospital's specialist department of child and adolescent mental health.

We were also taught more advanced general nursing procedures, demonstrated in the practical rooms by the sister tutors. Examples of the practical skills included the dressing of wounds, the removal of stitches and clips, and the management of intravenous infusions including blood transfusions. When we'd finished this block, all the second-year competencies that we'd been taught in the school were marked in our cross-charts. Once everything was completed, we were presented with our second-year caps – these had the all-important red stripe on them.

Now we were ready to go back on to the wards. Our first year already felt like a distant memory; we were second years now, with the confidence, knowledge and stripe on our caps to prove it. However, I wasn't going to be spending my first second-year experience on a ward. Instead, I was to spend the next eight weeks in the main theatres.

I had taken children to the suite of theatres on the sixth floor before, but only to the anaesthetic room. I'd never been in the theatres themselves, and a mixture of nerves and excitement bubbled up in me at the prospect. Once I had learnt the basics of theatre work, I was to be on the "twilight shift", which involved opening and setting up the theatre, then supporting the surgeon when a child needed an emergency operation outside daytime working hours. This meant having to uproot myself from my familiar room on the third floor of the nurses' home to one where I was more readily available and could be contacted by phone without disturbing anyone.

Before I began work on my first day in the theatres, I remembered to have a good breakfast as there was no way I was going to let myself down and faint. Once there, I met the very welcoming senior sister, who pressed a theatre manual into my hand.

"Lots for you to study there, Nurse," she said with a big smile. "General information about your duties and instructions on how you'll support staff during a routine operation."

"Thank you, Sister," I said, perfectly aware this would become my bible for the next few months.

She allocated me to one of the six theatres and introduced me to the staff nurse who was responsible for that theatre and would show me my morning duties.

My role every morning was to ensure that the surgeons' lockers contained the correct, clean operating clothes, and that the scrub room, where the surgeons and scrub nurse sanitised their hands and arms before the operation, had appropriate gowns and gloves available. I then had to go into the anaesthetic room, where the children were put to sleep. I had to open and test all the flow meters for gases that went to the machines in this room and in theatre, make sure that the suction worked and also ensure that all the necessary tubing and the correct sizes of catheters were available.

At the end of the day, when the operating lists had finished, I was responsible for checking all flow meters were turned off, any special apparatus (as well as pillows and blankets) were put away and, finally, that any used bowls and receivers left in the sluice were scrubbed in hot soapy water, dried and put in the autoclave for sterilisation.

For the first five weeks, I was to learn the role of the theatre runner. Before the operation, I (the runner) and the nurse who was assisting the surgeon (called the "scrub nurse"), counted all the swabs out loud from the sterile trolley and recorded the number on the theatre blackboard. At the end of the operation, as the wound was being stitched up, we counted the swabs again and again recorded them on the blackboard to make sure none had been retained in the wound.

During the operation, I had to be on hand to find anything extra that was needed by both the surgeon and the scrub nurse. I became confident in how to put on and dispose of my own cotton masks and disposable gloves, how to prevent contamination of sterile surfaces and instruments, how to sterilise instruments that were wanted quickly or dropped on the floor, as well as how to open and transfer anything sterile that was in a packet to the trolley and keep it sterile. During the operation, I also had to find time to prepare the trolley and instruments for the next case.

I had to learn by heart the names of the 16 different instruments available in a general theatre pack, which was used for routine procedures – including some instruments, such as dissecting forceps, of which we had more than one pair. I had to lay them out on the trolley in the order in which they were needed. This was so that when the surgeon asked for a particular instrument, the nurse who was scrubbed could hand it to him straight away without having to look through all the instruments to find the right one. It could then be returned to the correct place on the trolley after being used.

Finally, when the operation had finished, I took the used trolley and instruments into the sluice and, if necessary, mopped the theatre floor ready for the next case.

This routine was repeated for each operation. It was a lot to remember and I had to be on the ball.

The atmosphere in a theatre was very different to being on the ward. Creating a space in which the surgeons could focus completely was of the utmost importance. Some demanded absolute silence, such as James Crooks, the ENT surgeon. Others liked classical music playing in the background. At the end of surgery, they might chatter while stitching the wound as that didn't require so much concentration, but the real, more interesting chatter took place in the theatre restroom over coffee. I got to know the surgeons and staff very well.

I remember once being in the theatre while Mr Matthews, the consultant plastic surgeon, was operating. To my surprise, Mr Lloyd-Roberts, the orthopaedic surgeon from the theatre next door, walked in with his hands clasped in front of him so he couldn't contaminate them as he was scrubbed for his own operation. He was obviously killing time waiting for his next patient to arrive from his ward.

He peered over the wound that Mr Matthews was stitching. "How's the embroidery going then, David?" he asked seriously.

The theatre erupted into laughter. It was well known that orthopaedic surgeons would stitch a wound together using about five stitches while a plastic surgeon would use up to fifteen.

At the end of six weeks, I had to have learnt which instruments were in the packs for a hernia operation and a removal of the appendix. I knew the types of tissue and names of the muscles that were divided during these operations. I knew the different needles used to repair both muscles and skin so that I could hand the right threaded needle or forceps to the surgeon at the right time.

The reason I had to learn all this was that, after taking a written test, I had to "scrub" and assist the surgeon in the operation myself. The staff nurse observed my competence as a "scrub nurse" and gave me feedback on how well I performed during the removal of an appendix. I enjoyed the experience. The surgeon I scrubbed for was patient with me and praised me at the end of the procedure.

Working in the theatre was fast-paced and fascinating, juggling many responsibilities and remembering huge amounts of information. What I had missed was building strong relationships with the children – it's hard to bond with them when they are asleep!

My first ward in my second year was 3A&B, a medical ward. One side was devoted to children with skin problems and the other was mixed medical. This year, instead of the sluice, we were responsible for the treatment room. This was an area where children would come for minor procedures, so the setting up of the room and the trolleys were now familiar to me.

On the wards, unlike in the theatres, we had no theatre packs made up in the hospital sterile department. Everything we used came from autoclaved (steam sterilising) drums. Trolleys had to be laid up using long-handled "Cheatle forceps", which took practice to use. Picking up an instrument from the drum without dropping it was deceptively challenging!

There were also no pre-packed dressings. All of these had to be made and packed into a drum by us students. (This would surprise staff today.) If we had a slack time on any ward, a large roll of gauze had to be cut up and folded into squares to use as dressings. Similarly, a large roll of cotton wool would have to be made into balls for cleaning wounds. These were then packed into the drum and sent for autoclaving. Occasionally I witnessed a staff nurse helping with this task. None of us was ever allowed to be idle.

We'd do our best to distract the children in the treatment room by using toys. We'd be as quick and efficient as possible, but they still didn't like visiting the treatment room as it normally meant injections, taking blood or putting in a cannula to give an intravenous infusion of blood or other fluids. Later, when parents were allowed to stay with their child, it was easier – not that they were ever happy when their child was upset, but they could comfort them better than us.

Another role for the second-year student was to assist in the giving out of medicines with a staff nurse. The drug cupboard contained routine prescription medicines. A second locked cupboard inside the main cupboard contained the "controlled drugs". These were – and still are – under strict government regulation because they could be addictive or misused. Two members of staff, one of whom had to be a registered sick children's trained nurse, checked the controlled medicines.

Although measuring and recording the dose of a medicine was always of huge importance, it was even more so when using the controlled medicines. Signing to say that these had been given was made on the prescription chart and also in the controlled drug book. The amounts used and remaining in the cupboard were checked daily by staff.

This procedure hasn't changed over the years. It is important today that these medicines aren't mislaid or stolen. Once any medicine was checked, the two staff checking it went to the bedside together with the prescription and medicine on a tray and checked the armband of the child, making sure the name and hospital number of the child were the same as on the prescription chart. The junior staff member was then left at the bedside to make sure that the child took the medicine. This wasn't always easy if the medicine tasted horrible or were tablets that had to be crushed and disguised in a spoonful of jam. Our responsibilities were growing day by day.

My friend, Patricia, had begun her three-year training before me. In her first year on her second ward experience, there was a leaking tap in the sluice. Her ward sister, who was infamously formidable, instructed Patricia to look out for the plumber and show him to the sluice and the leaking tap. Patricia spotted a gentleman coming on to the ward in an old raincoat, carrying a holdall. She swooped, gathered him up and led him to the sluice. She showed him the offending tap and gave him a quick tour of the sluice. He expressed great interest and gave the impression that this was the first time he had seen inside a sluice, somewhat bizarre for a hospital plumber.

"Nurse," thundered her ward sister. "Why have you brought my consultant into the sluice?"

The consultant giggled. "I've never had so much fun," he said.

Patricia was forgiven.

There's a sequel to this story. Patricia's father was himself a consultant at another hospital. When he was at home one day having lunch with his family, a young surgeon joined them. During the meal he regaled them with one of his father's experiences.

His father was a consultant at Great Ormond Street and was visiting his ward one day. A young student nurse had mistaken him for the plumber and given him a tour of the sluice. He described the tour in detail. An embarrassed Patricia owned up before the story continued for too long!

Ward 3A&B was a good place for teaching students, as it had a number of babies in the side wards. While I was on the skin side of the ward, several babies there had severe eczema. We had to soak these babies every morning for 20 minutes in a bath of emulsifying ointment solution – this is a long time to entertain a baby in a bath. I enjoyed giving this treatment as it made my hands feel wonderfully soft. We then had to slather the baby's skin with prescription creams using disposable gloves.

There were some very sad cases of unpleasant skin conditions. A little girl, Sally, was on the ward for most of my experience on 3A&B. Her skin was so fragile that any friction caused large blisters and wounds to form. She had sores all round her face and on her fingernails from where she touched her face and sucked her fingers. She wore a very cool, loose dress and was handled as little as possible, and then only by senior staff, but she was very vocal in letting her needs be known. Every morning, she stood in her cot, shouting to be taken out of her cubicle and put in her beloved ward pram.

Sally's morning bath had emulsifying ointment and added salt, but she wouldn't stay as long in it as the other children. Afterwards, her skin would be moisturised well to stop her scratching, and the sore areas were treated with prescription ointments and non-stick paraffin gauze dressings. The worst sores were in her elbow and knee joints. Although she slept and was cared for in a side room, she completely lit up around the other children in the playroom. She couldn't play with them, but some of them got to know her. They knew they couldn't touch her, but they would offer her toys to play with. She loved attention and got a lot of it, particularly from the staff.

On the general medical side of the ward, we nursed children's blood disorders. Children with haemophilia, which affects the blood's ability to clot, were admitted regularly. If these children fell over and hurt themselves enough to cause prolonged bleeding and/or severe bruising, they had to come into hospital for a transfusion of plasma. Plasma contains platelets, which help the blood to clot. These children were also given anti-haemophiliac globulin containing factor VIII, as they were deficient in this.[11] This gave them relief for a short while until they hurt themselves again. Today, patients or their parents can manage haemophilia at home with regular injections of factor VIII.

Another blood disorder I remember nursing was sickle cell anaemia, which is particularly common in families of African or Caribbean descent. Children start showing symptoms of this disease during the first year of their life, often when they're around five months old. These children make red blood cells that are "sickle" shaped. These cells die sooner than healthy cells, causing the child to have fewer red cells in their blood, making them anaemic.[13] They too were admitted to our ward for regular blood transfusions.

An interesting fact about this condition is that when sickle cells give up their oxygen to the tissues, they stick together, forming long rods inside the red blood cells. This makes them rigid and sickle shaped.[14] These cells cannot squeeze through small blood vessels, so the vessels get blocked and cause the child pain.

The children on our ward often complained of pain in their fingers and swelling in their toes, but the only medicines we could give them were folic acid, which triggered the production of new red blood cells, and painkillers to ease the pain.[13] In the 1960s, sickle cell disease was only seen in children, with few children ever reaching adulthood. Today, although people live longer with this disease, the only cure involves having stem cell or bone marrow transplants.

In the early 1960s, the giving of blood was a very time-consuming exercise and something that I had to learn, as it was done regularly on 3A&B. There was a strict protocol for collecting and managing blood before it was given to a child.

After I was shown the aseptic technique of putting the intravenous line into the blood bag and connecting it to the tube that went into the child's arm, I had to regulate the flow of blood by hand. There were no machines to do this. Blood dripped into a chamber halfway down the line (this is why patients call it their "drip"), and this was controlled by a roller clamp on the tube. Using a formula, I worked out how many drips per minute would give the measured amount of blood that was prescribed.

Every quarter of an hour, I would check that the drip rate was right, counting the drips while looking at my watch, altering the flow if necessary and charting how much blood had been given to the child. The roller clamp wasn't easy to control and it could take a number of minutes to get right. It really was a hands-on, intensive job. Giving too much blood could damage the child's heart, so it was so important to get it right.

Giving transfusions to children with blood disorders regularly helped me to learn about the different types of blood and blood products. I was also taught the very strict protocols for the management of blood within the hospital, including how to collect blood from the blood bank and store it for a short period on the ward, and the double-checking of the blood before it was given to the child.

I'd started on 3A&B in December and Christmas was fast approaching. I was asked if I would be Angel Gabriel in the hospital nativity play and, knowing how much fun it had been in the previous year, I agreed. It meant rehearsing in my off-duty time, which at least excused me from painting the cubicle and ward windows, as my artistic skills hadn't improved.

This Christmas Eve, some of our set was invited to the traditional visit to Covent Garden Market. It was still very much thriving in those days, even though the Covent Garden Market Bill had been passed in 1961 – to relocate the market as it was so congested. By 1974, it had moved in its entirety to Nine Elms across the river. But for now, I was very excited to be a part of this annual outing to collect fruit and veg for GOS.

We left the hospital discreetly but in uniform wearing our capes. Christmas in London is a magical time and we wanted to give the children as much of this as possible – as did the stall holders. It was a bustling place, full of colour and noise and delightful smells, with flowers, roasting chestnuts, oranges and lemons. There were lights and decorations and a massive Christmas tree. Customers jostled and queued for last-minute bargains. Barrow boys dodged wooden crates and pallets with their trolleys. Porters were rushing around carrying barrels and baskets on their heads. The stall holders all recognised us, knowing we'd come from the children's hospital. They handed over bags and even boxes of fruit, flowers and vegetables.

"This is for the kids, God bless 'em."

When we'd collected much more than we could carry, the police took us back to the hospital. The tradition was that they brought a Black Mariah to collect us and our spoils. This was a large police van with two wooden benches along each side below high barred windows. It was used not only to carry prisoners but also large groups of police if they were needed for street disturbances. The police locked us in this van, and we acted the part.

"Let me out! Let me out!" we would shout, banging on the side of the vehicle to heighten the drama. Doing so was a key part of the tradition and never failed to have us falling about laughing.

On Christmas Day on the ward, every member of staff was present. As usual, no one was allowed home. Sally was in her element. A member of staff had found her a lovely loose cotton dress with embroidered pintucks across the front. To top it all off, she'd also been made a crown of tinsel, which sat proudly on her head.

Yet again, some poor member of the medical staff had taken on the important role of Father Christmas and came up the hospital drive in a sleigh surrounded by elves. We took Sally, and other children that we were able to get on to the balcony, to wave and cheer at the procession as it passed us and entered the hospital. Sally was so excited at the thought of the presents Father Christmas would bring her, she could hardly contain herself. Various other medical staff had already been press-ganged into dressing up as Santa; it was too big a job for one man to give out presents to all the children on the 17 wards. Of course, there would always be one vigilant child who noticed that the Father Christmas who gave him his present was different from the one who came up the drive. That was a tricky thing to explain.

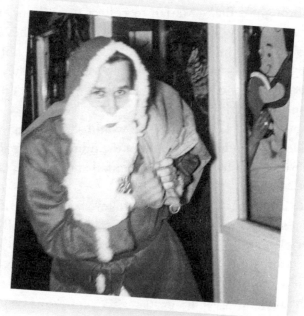

3A&B's Father Christmas.

Our Christmas Day lunch was well organised on 3A&B. The turkey was carved by the senior registrar as the consultant physician was on holiday.

Christmas Day and Boxing Day were very relaxing and the food was excellent. We were even allowed one glass of wine as a special treat. Unfortunately we didn't have this respite for long and our normal working hours resumed as soon as Christmas was over.

PATIENT CARE STUDY

During our second-year teaching block, we were asked to start thinking about a child who might be suitable for our next patient care study. Jeremy, the young lad with tetanus, had been my first, so I wondered who to do this year. Eventually I decided on a young girl I had nursed on 7CD, which meant returning to the ENT ward to get more information about her.

Vicky was admitted to hospital with noisy breathing when she was a day old. It was during her stay there that she developed a chest infection and became very ill. She recovered well from the infection following antibiotics, but still had noisy breathing. The ENT surgeon at her hospital diagnosed her as having a non-cancerous lesion (an abnormal change in the tissue) and asked Mr Crooks (our ENT surgeon) to take over her care.

Vicky was first admitted to GOS before her first birthday for the removal of this lesion, which took a number of attempts to remove completely. The lesion lay just above her voice box, which meant it was not only difficult to remove, but it was also difficult for the anaesthetist to put her to sleep for the operation. At each operation, Vicky had a tracheostomy. During one of the operations, the anaesthetist had to place the tube for the anaesthetic gases through the tracheostomy opening to allow more space for Mr Crooks to work.

Vicky recovered remarkably well from these operations and was eventually discharged completely from the care of GOS but with a letter from the hospital to be shown to any doctor who she might see in the future. This letter recorded details of Vicky's past breathing problems and the operations she had undergone.

Later, as a young girl, Vicky developed a persistent cough and wheezing after having whooping cough. She was admitted to her local hospital as she had great difficulty in speaking. There they examined Vicky's larynx under anaesthetic and took a biopsy of a small swelling, which they thought was cancerous. Vicky was transferred to GOS for a second opinion.

This was when I met Vicky – when she was admitted to 7CD. Her mother was very anxious about her, but fortunately talked freely about her concerns. She told us about Vicky's cough, which was worse at night and had been particularly bad for the past week, with her coughing spasms lasting up to five minutes.

"She coughs so much that she wheezes and chokes," she said, clearly distressed. "She seems to stop breathing and goes all blue. It's terrifying."

Vicky's mum also told us how worried she was about the possibility of a cancer diagnosis and hoped that this would not be found at GOS.

Vicky, on the other hand, appeared to have no worries. Although she had difficulty with breathing and her voice was very husky, she actually enjoyed being in hospital and explored everything we kept for children in the playroom.

"I love reading," she said. "Especially adventure stories."

She examined all the books we had – *The Famous Five* and *Secret Seven*, *Paddington Bear* and *Swallows and Amazons*. She told me that she had read many of them already. I could see that Vicky enjoyed these adventure stories, as many of our young girls did. They took her off on a flight of fancy, but she still very much liked being a part of life on the ward.

She quickly made friends with a girl of a similar age to her. What the two of them enjoyed most was watching the babies on the ward being fed. The two girls would stand glued to the cubicle windows, taking in everything that the staff were doing for the babies.

"I'd love to get married when I grow up," Vicky whispered to me one day.

"And why is that, Vicky?" I asked her.

"Because I want to be a mummy," she answered.

Before Vicky went for surgery, she had lots of tests and observations, all of which were normal. We were to observe her coughing attacks, which were exactly as her mother described and really were quite frightening to watch, even though Vicky took them in her stride. As soon as an attack subsided, she'd say she was fine and carry on as normal.

The medical staff tried to control her coughing with a medicine used to treat allergic reactions. This also had a sedative effect. It did reduce the intensity of her coughing fits, but Vicky continued to speak with her husky voice. The time came for Mr Crooks to examine her larynx under anaesthetic and take another biopsy for the laboratory to test.

Vicky was her normal calm and very practical self when we prepared her for theatre. As she was on the morning list, she couldn't have food after midnight but was allowed to drink up until four hours before it was time to go. For this last drink, as was usual, we gave Vicky a glass of water with a teaspoon of glucose powder dissolved in it, to make sure she maintained a good level of sugar in her blood. Vicky was very happy to read one of our books, which she hadn't read before, until it was time for her premedication, which was prescribed an hour and a half before she was due to go to theatre.

A premedication was always given in the 1960s before a child went to theatre. It was a sedative combined with a medicine to dry up the fluid in the mouth and throat to make the operation site easier to view. It was given by injection into the child's backside, which they didn't like, but was done so swiftly and expertly by GOS staff that the child hardly knew they'd had it.

Paediatric nurses were very experienced at giving injections. It was a competency that the sister tutors and registered staff were very insistent that we should do well. Giving an injection badly can not only cause pain and damage to the surrounding tissue, but also destroys the confidence of the child for having any procedure done in hospital. We'd prepared Vicky for having this injection and, when it came to having it, she made no fuss at all.

Vicky's mother and we nurses were very anxious to know what Mr Crooks would find in theatre. We hoped that there would not be any cancer cells, but we realised that only the laboratory report could confirm this. When Vicky returned to the ward, her mum was told by Mr Crooks that he found scarring of the vocal cords, as well as other small irregularities that he believed were normal scar tissue. There was one small swelling that he biopsied, but he thought that it was just scar tissue as well.

The biopsy report was sent through from the laboratory the following day. The microscopic examination showed cells that were similar to those seen on Vicky's previous biopsy eight years ago. There was no sign of cancer. This was a normal result with normal tissue found. We were all very relieved, especially Vicky's mother. Vicky knew nothing about the suspected diagnosis so was unaware of our concerns.

Vicky was discharged home with her antihistamine medicines for her gradually improving cough. Her mum was warned that Vicky's voice might continue to be slightly husky as she had scar tissue on her vocal cords from the operation as a baby. Her mum was so relieved that Vicky didn't have cancer, she felt they could cope with that. It was such a good outcome.

I was approaching my period of night duty in my second year. This time I would be taking more responsibility on the ward and would be being tested on my management skills. I was to work on 5E, the burns unit in the central block of the hospital. The ward had six cubicles and was isolated from the main wards.

While I was here, five boys aged between 10 and 12 were admitted with severe burns. They had broken into a disused factory and opened a fuse box, which promptly exploded. All of them had burns to their faces and the upper part of their bodies. Three were very badly burnt and barely conscious. They were all isolated, each in their own cubicle, and barrier-nursed to reduce the risk of infection.

I'd never seen anyone with severe burns, but knew that children with bad burns could die of shock, so this was the first thing to treat. Back then, oxygen was given by erecting an oxygen tent over patients. The medical staff spent a frantic time trying to find veins that would take an intravenous line so we could give the boys essential fluids to minimise the effects of shock. We were so busy that extra staff had been brought in to help on the unit. We were working on a combination of adrenaline and auto pilot.

We had to calculate the amount of fluid to give to each child. This amount depended on accurately calculating the surface area and depth of the burnt areas.[15] We had charts to help us calculate this. The younger the child, the bigger percentage their head was to the rest of their body. Then we added the depth of the burns, classified into five degrees, with the fifth degree being the deepest.[16] I remember the calculations being between 25 and 40 per cent of these children's bodies. We knew it was possible that none of them would survive.

The children had to have a catheter inserted into their bladders, as measuring their fluid output and intake was very important. They also had antibiotics to try to prevent infection, another cause of death in patients with severe burns. One child had to have a tracheostomy to help him breathe.

We were so focused on our work that we had no time to dwell on the horrific results of these boys' actions. I later learnt that, tragically, one of them died. Those who did survive were specialled for a number of weeks. Not only were they monitored closely, but they had to go to the operating theatre for debridement (removal of dead tissue from their wounds) and for skin grafts to help with healing.

I was too junior to do any specialling, but I was assisting in many procedures that were new to me. I was managing oxygen, performing catheter care, emptying the urine drainage bags, improving my ability to perform aseptic technique by changing wound dressings and at long last removing stitches. I was also having a lot of practice giving injections into muscles. These children were in our care, and it was our duty to do everything we could to preserve their lives. Sadly, despite our very best efforts, we couldn't always achieve that.

Despite the lows, there were moments of fun. During this block of night duty, in a rare moment of quiet, one of us might make some chocolate cornflakes in the ward kitchen. It became tradition to ring a friend you knew was busy and tell them you were about to send some up in the lift. Because I was very busy with these boys, Carol rang me one night.

"I'm sending you a plate," she told me.

"Thanks, Carol," I said. "You're a pal."

I could picture her putting the plate of chocolate cornflakes on the floor of the lift and pressing the button for the fifth floor to send them on their way. We always hoped and prayed that no one would intercept the lift on the way, particularly Matron. I then listened out for the old lift rattling up the floors. It was easy to know when it had arrived and I could quickly retrieve the goodies. I shared them with the staff nurse who was specialling the boy with the tracheostomy and they certainly lifted our spirits. In those days, I think it was the most daring thing we students ever got up to. We'd never have done it in our first year, so this shows we must definitely have been growing in confidence.

After our three months of night duty, we were always ready for a break and this, thankfully, was the time that our two-week holiday was due. The first week of my holiday was spent at home in my grandmother's house, just south of Hammersmith Bridge.

My family were still living with her in a flat in the upstairs part of the house. My brother was now nine and my sister would soon be three. My mother ran a private physiotherapy practice from the house when I was small, but with two young children she'd had to put this on the back burner. Later, she worked rehabilitating elderly patients following serious illnesses or strokes, helping them return to independent living.

Our Alsatian dog, Sarah, would hear me coming home and would get excited even before I'd opened the front gate. She would jump all over me, licking my face and then follow me everywhere I went.

My grandmother was now 78 and as active and independent as ever. Every Sunday, she would cook herself a full roast dinner with a joint, roast potatoes and vegetables. She even made her own gravy. The joint would be sliced up for meals to last her the rest of the week. I remember that as a child my treat was to sit with her at her kitchen table, eating toast with lashings of butter (rationed during and after the war) and Marmite. She had a daily routine of cleaning and laying the coal fires and a weekly routine of doing her washing and cleaning all the brass in the house, including the brass letter box and the knocker on the front door. I was always very thrilled to see my grandmother, who would be waiting with bated breath for a blow-by-blow account of everything I'd been doing over the last few months.

During the second week, Carol, another student from our set, Judy and I went to the Lake District. We spent a few exhausting days youth hostelling, hitch-hiking and clambering up hills. We certainly had fun. We felt perfectly safe doing this, though looking back, Carol remarked to me, "How irresponsible was that?!"

I then went with Carol to her home in Todmorden in Yorkshire. Carol had two brothers and, like my friend Carol from school, her brothers got up to mischief. Carol remembers one morning one of her brothers and a cousin of theirs lighting a fire in the open fireplace in their living room. I don't know what they used as an accelerant for the fire, but they set the chimney alight. As Carol was still in her pyjamas, I was sent with the boys to the nearest phone box to ring the fire brigade. Her mother was not pleased when she returned home and unjustly blamed Carol for not keeping an eye on them.

THE END OF SECOND YEAR

Before my group could go on to our adult hospital for our third year of training, I had to go back to GOS and my two final wards. Both of them were medical wards.

The first ward was 5C&D, where I met Professor Moncrieff face to face. He was the consultant paediatrician and professor in child health, who had taught us about common medical conditions in the School of Nursing. What he hadn't told us was that he was doing a research study on children with suspected lead poisoning. Apparently the condition was well recognised and common in the United States and they had found evidence that lead poisoning in children resulted in them having emotional and intellectual difficulties.

The condition hadn't been recognised previously in the UK, but methods for determining levels of lead in the blood were becoming more freely available, so Professor Moncrieff had been admitting children who'd been given a preliminary diagnosis of encephalitis (inflammation of the brain) by other physicians. He was also admitting children referred to him with unexplained anaemia, behavioural and developmental problems, convulsions, unexplained abdominal pain, vomiting and changes in their behaviour. All these children were having blood tests for lead levels and other detailed investigations to check for lead poisoning.

Professor Moncrieff was particularly interested in these children's living conditions, the trade of the father and the behaviour of the child at home. Of the 20 children who were part of the research from January 1961 to May 1963, five came from excellent homes, both economically and socially. Twelve of the families lived in unfavourable conditions – poorly maintained old flats or tenement buildings, mostly with unsatisfactory means of rubbish disposal. These children had to be removed from their home and the source of the lead by being admitted to hospital, while the local health authority searched for lead in the home and surrounding environment. This sometimes led to a medical recommendation for the family to be rehoused.

It wasn't always clear how these children accessed the lead, but there was often opportunity. For instance, one patient was the child of a carpenter and played with putty containing red lead. Others chewed the bars of their cot or outside railings. Another child's father paint-sprayed cars when the child was present. Another family grew vegetables on soil containing numerous lead battery casings from an old electricity-generating plant. Samples of cabbages from their allotment and blood from all the family members showed high levels of lead. Other children who were affected were in the habit of eating non-nutritious items or harmful substances such as paper, hair, stones and soil.[17]

The collection of blood samples was one of the most important diagnostic tests for lead poisoning but, as lead remained in the blood for around 36 days, it was only an indicator of recent exposure.[18] Other tests included X-rays to examine for lead particles in the gut and, if a diagnosis couldn't be confirmed by these methods, taking a bone marrow sample for analysis. These were the main places where lead would be stored in the child's body.

These children were observed carefully, particularly those with abdominal pain and vomiting who may have chewed on painted objects or swallowed something with a high lead content. As lead is carried in the red blood cells and stops oxygen from getting to the brain, we were also recording any unexplained behaviour patterns these children might have. Lead would also be found in the bowel and, as it would persist here for long periods of time, we removed it by performing enemas, at which I was becoming quite competent.

Any child diagnosed with lead poisoning would be treated with medicines to remove the lead from their blood and tissues. These medicines were called chelating agents and bound the metal to them, enabling the medicine to be discharged safely from the body in the child's urine. There were two different medicines – one given by mouth for milder cases of lead poisoning and another by injection into muscles or, in severe cases, into a vein.

We were responsible for collecting all urine from these children and sending each collection to the laboratory daily to evaluate the lead output to prove that the medicines were working. Within a month of treatment, some parents noticed a marked improvement in both their child's behaviour and social development.[17] It was a remarkable result.

The research of Professor Moncrieff and his team concluded that children with a high lead content in their blood had some brain and central nervous system problems. This was a very positive outcome with far-reaching consequences for the health of children and their families, underlining the importance of clinical studies at GOS. At the end of 1963, a voluntary agreement was made between what was then the Paintmakers Association of Great Britain (now the British Coatings Federation) and the UK government – that if paint contained more than 1 per cent of lead, then its label should provide a warning that the paint should not be applied to surfaces accessible to children.[19]

It wasn't until some 30 years later (in 1992) that the banning of lead in household paint came into effect, as well as the limiting of the concentration of lead in food. It was the result of EU legislation and was implemented in the UK under the Controls on Injurious Substances Regulations.[19]

The other experience I had on 5CD was the care of children with growth problems who were being monitored on regular intramuscular injections of growth hormone. Growth hormone is made by a gland that lies deep within the brain. Any problems with this gland, or with the instructions sent to it, may stop children growing properly. The slowing down of a child's growth is usually picked up from the age of two years onwards. Although children with growth hormone deficiency grow in proportion, they grow less than other children and are much shorter when they reach adulthood. Some women may be as much as eight inches shorter than a woman who grows normally.[20] There's also the risk that puberty may happen later than usual or not occur at all.

I remember one nine-year-old girl called Edna. She was on growth hormone therapy, and she made friends with another nine-year-old called Janet, who was of normal size. They were inseparable and Janet was very protective of Edna. We had to push their beds in the ward next to each other, they had to have their meals in the playroom together and they both loved dancing.

My final ward in my second year was 3C&D. This was also a medical ward. It was here that I met again the young boy who'd been diagnosed at 18 months with type 1 diabetes on Cohen Ward. He was admitted for stabilisation and reassessment. His character had remained delightful; he was full of smiles and loved by all the staff.

The ward also treated children with respiratory problems. We had children with asthma, who were either diagnosed at the hospital or admitted during an asthma attack and given nebulisers and antibiotics to treat an infection. Because we didn't have an accident and emergency department, the parents of children whose asthma was difficult to control had yellow cards, which would allow them to return to the hospital in an emergency and gain access to the ward. These children would be treated, re-stabilised on their inhalers and sent home when they were well enough.

I remember nursing a child with croup (noisy breathing and a cough), who was given steam inhalations. He was about six months old and confined to his cot. We used a kettle to fill his cubicle with steam. The health and safety issues were enormous. The kettle was erected in a corner of the cubicle well away from his cot. Only nursing and medical staff could enter the cubicle, and then under strict safety guidelines. But it was well worth the trouble as it was so effective at easing his symptoms.

Steam inhalations were used all the time on this ward. It was one of the treatments for cystic fibrosis. Cystic fibrosis is an inherited condition that causes sticky mucus to build up in the lungs and digestive system. Babies suspected of having this disease were admitted for tests immediately. Their first symptom would be malnutrition; the lung problems would start later.

In the 1940s and earlier, children with cystic fibrosis died of malnutrition due to clogging of the pancreas with mucus, which affected their digestion of food. In 1948, Dr Paul di Sant'Agnese, who was observing babies who were sick with dehydration during a New York heat wave, discovered they had abnormally high concentrations of salt in their sweat. This led to the development of the "sweat test", which is still used to diagnose cystic fibrosis today.[21]

Babies diagnosed with cystic fibrosis need regular follow-up appointments and treatment to help control the symptoms. Even now, there's no cure for this condition. Pancreatic enzyme and vitamin supplements, as well as a high-calorie diet, would help to prevent malnutrition. Unfortunately, the pancreatic enzyme tablets were large, oval, brown things that tasted and smelt disgusting. The children were *not* happy to take them, and jam could only disguise so much.

Steam inhalations and physiotherapy were used to remove mucus from the lungs in addition to antibiotics to treat chest infections. As children became older and developed lung problems, the steam inhalations were given to them in steam tents while they slept at night. This loosened the mucus before their twice-daily physiotherapy. Children were beginning to survive until their early teens with these treatments, but it's telling that I was marked as competent at "last offices" on this ward. I'd never felt less happy to have a competency checked off.

I remember a baby born with Pierre Robin syndrome, as it was known then. This condition was first defined by Pierre Robin in 1923.[22] He described babies who were born with a lower jaw that hadn't grown, a tongue set back in the mouth, and difficulty breathing. In a later publication Robin added a cleft palate (a gap in the roof of the mouth) to this condition.[23/24] The presence of the tongue positioned at the back of the mouth was believed to have caused this U-shaped gap in the baby's palate when he or she was in the womb.

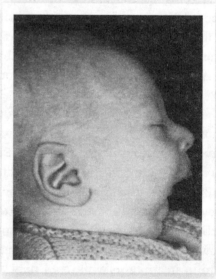

A three-week-old baby with a small jaw.

Much later, in the early 2000s, I worked with babies born with a small jaw. I remember examining them as newborns and observing the position of their tongue, which was firmly wedged in the cleft of their palate. This caused an obstruction, which resulted in breathing problems that could become life-threatening. They were immediately transferred to our specialist unit to manage their breathing and feeding. In the 1960s, methods of improving the breathing of these children had mainly been either to stitch the tongue to the floor of the mouth,[25] or, as an emergency measure, to give these babies a tracheostomy. Medical staff tried to avoid this latter, drastic operation on a newborn. Neither of these methods helped the child with their feeding.

On Ward 3C&D, I observed a baby with this condition being nursed on a special cradle. Bromley and Burston (from the Royal Liverpool Children's Hospital in Heswall on the Wirral) had observed that the tongue of these babies would fall forward easily if they were nursed in the correct position. Burston, a consultant orthodontist, developed this special cradle on which the babies could be nursed facing downwards, which would allow both their jaw and the tongue to hang forward.

Burston wrote, "The normal routine would be for a child to be nursed for two hours on and one hour off the frame for a period of two to three months." He concluded, "during this period the jaw would have grown forward considerably."[26]

On 3C&D, the baby I was observing, who we will call Peter, was having a trial on this cradle to avoid an operation. It consisted of a plaster shell mounted on a frame, which was fitted over the lowered bars of his cot. Peter lay on the frame on his front with his face through a hole. Below this hole, a mirror lay on the bed to allow easy observation of his jaw and tongue.

Normally, a baby learns and practises the skills of sucking and swallowing by drinking his mother's amniotic fluid in the womb, but this isn't possible if their tongue is wedged in the cleft of the palate. Peter was born unable to feed instinctively and too weak to learn to nourish himself because of his breathing difficulties. He also had a weak suck due to his cleft. His situation at birth had been life-threatening, so breastfeeding wasn't possible, but we encouraged Peter's mother to express her milk, which contained her antibodies, so we could give this to him by bottle.

Encouraging Peter to learn the skills of feeding was very important, so he was taken off the cradle to be fed using a bottle with a long teat, lying on his side on one of his parents' or a nurse's lap. At first, Peter was too exhausted to take his full quota of feed, so a small tube, placed through his nose and into his stomach, gave any remaining feed. While he was nursed on the Burston cradle, Peter was not only being taught to feed properly, but he was also learning to control his tongue and to protect his airway. After three months, he was considered to be out of danger.[26] During this period, Peter's parents had also been learning to care for him. Once they were confident to do this, he was able to go home.

When he was 15 months, Peter's weight was satisfactory for his age and he was getting used to a normal diet.[27] He was now ready for the next stage of his treatment. He was admitted to 4C&D, the plastic surgery ward under Mr Matthews, to have his cleft palate closed.

While I was on 4C&D, I saw many children who'd been operated on for a repair of a cleft palate. Mr Matthews would realign the soft palate muscles so the child could develop normal speech. The operation was even more traumatic for

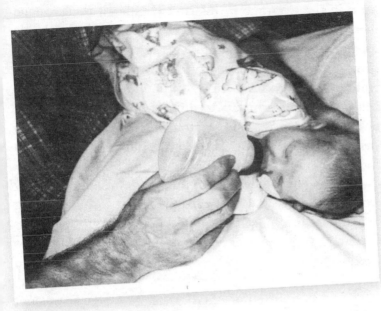

Peter's father learning to feed him.

the child in those days than it is now. Cuts in the palate were made on each side of the cleft and packed with antiseptic gauze. Peter would have returned from theatre with a stitch in the back of his tongue which, if necessary, could be pulled forward to open his airway. He would also return with splints on his arms, made out of cardboard rolls, to stop him from putting his fingers in his mouth. Today, the operation is done at a younger age with improved techniques and the children recover more quickly from this drastic surgery.

Peter would have been sent home after his packs were removed. He would then have been seen every six months in the outpatient clinic by Mr Matthews, who monitored the progress of his speech development. At the age of five, if deemed necessary, he'd be referred to a speech and language therapist.[27] Today, the speech and language therapist is present with the consultant surgeon in the outpatient clinics after the operation, and the two of them assess the child's speech together.

As for me, my time at Great Ormond Street was coming to a close for now. It was a strange feeling. Not only was the work so stimulating and exciting, but I truly felt like I'd found a home there. Now I was looking forward to a new experience, training with adults.

THIRD YEAR:
HAMMERSMITH HOSPITAL

After our third-year teaching block, during which we consolidated our learning about adult diseases, I went to Hammersmith Hospital along with five other students from my set for our practical experience. We wore our pink-and-white uniform, as was usual for GOS nurses when working elsewhere. We were proud to do this, especially now we had our strings cap, knowing we'd be recognised and respected as GOS nurses.

Hammersmith Hospital also has an interesting history. Since its establishment in the early twentieth century on a large area of open space known as Wormwood Scrubs, it's been a smallpox hospital, a workhouse and infirmary, an orthopaedic military hospital and a tuberculosis (TB) dispensary. The infirmary's impressive building was once known as "the Palace on the Scrubs" as so much money had been spent on it but, by the time we arrived there, some of the ward blocks were in dire need of upgrading.

It was a large, busy hospital known for its pioneering treatment and research for patients who were in kidney failure. It had a renowned kidney dialysis and transplant unit that began the first haemodialysing in the UK in 1947 (a way of removing waste material and poisons from the blood of these patients). There was a reason why renal (kidney) expertise was developed here; it was as a result of the Second World War.

Since the hospital was situated just outside central London, it received many casualties dug out of bombed buildings at a late stage, often suffering from crush injuries. Many of these went on to have kidney failure. The effects of "crush syndrome and kidney failure" were published in 1941.[28] But Hammersmith Hospital was often in the news for quite a different reason. Its next-door neighbour was Wormwood Scrubs Prison.

For the first few months, we lived in the nurses' home, which was very close to the Scrubs. In fact, my room was overlooked by the long-stay wing, where most of the prisoners were in for lengthy sentences. There was a large notice behind the wardrobe door of each nurse's bedroom with the instruction "Do NOT undress without closing the curtains". One evening, without thinking and because it was rubbing my neck, I undid the starched collar of my dress as I walked into my room. I immediately saw lights flashing from the windows of the prison block. I drew my curtains quickly. There was no next time.

Sometimes even prisoners have to come into hospital. It wasn't uncommon to see inmates on a ward handcuffed to a prison officer, but this wasn't always foolproof. One prisoner was reputed to have escaped from a toilet window on the third floor down a drainpipe. If any prisoner tried to escape from the prison, the hospital was the first place to be searched. Once or twice the police actually invaded our dining room with sniffer dogs, hunting under all the tables while we were eating.

The six of us from GOS decided it would be better to rent a place together. These would be my new friends for the next year. There was Maggie, Penny, Anne, Debbie and Meg. We found a house in Putney within commuting distance of the hospital, which wasn't actually in Hammersmith but nearer to White City and Shepherd's Bush. Putney was quite an affluent area with lots of young families. As we had little money, we decided to offer our services locally as babysitters. We put an advertisement in the local paper shop saying that we were in our third year of training at the Hospital for Sick Children, Great Ormond Street, and would be available to babysit in the evenings. There was usually one of the six of us free each evening, so it became a practical and enjoyable way of making some extra cash.

The whole of our training at the Hammersmith was so much more relaxed than we were used to. My first ward, a male medical ward, was quite a baptism of fire. Nursing adult men was *not* like nursing children, and I really wasn't used to the banter that went back and forth. I remember a young man who was bed bound. I had drawn the bed curtains around him and was fetching a bowl of water for him to wash. He was stripped naked when I returned.

"I'd like a bed bath, Nurse," he said, winking at me.

I soaked his flannel in the water and threw it across his chest.

"Just get on with washing yourself," I said and walked away. I had learnt from GOS not to accept any nonsense from naughty little boys.

I remember a young man who was very poorly with cirrhosis of the liver (death and scarring of the liver cells).

"I'm dying from drink, Nurse," he admitted to me one day.

I was taken aback by his openness and humbled to witness his two neighbours determinedly making the last days of his life as cheerful as possible. Patients were allowed alcohol in the hospital if it was prescribed and given out on the medicine round but, even though these two patients weren't entitled to any, they made up for this by rioting every time there were no senior staff around.

One of the men, who was in for tests, didn't appear at all ill when he jumped from bed to bed, as if he were a boy – not that we would have tolerated such raucous behaviour from the boys back at GOS. Both he and his companion posed for my camera shots with inappropriate ward equipment, which would have given Miss Kirkby a heart attack. It probably wouldn't have impressed the matron of this hospital either if she'd known, but it really did lift the spirits of the dying young man.

I found the staff cared a lot for their patients. They were particularly concerned about an adult with learning disabilities, whom they appeared to know very well. They took a lot of trouble with him. This aspect of the hospital, and this ward in particular, impressed me. The high jinks certainly didn't prevent me from learning.

Provisions had been made for us to do our competencies here, just as we had done back at GOS when looking after children. I'd already learnt many of the tasks, such as performing dressings, giving oxygen, passing a tube through the nose and into the stomach to give liquid food

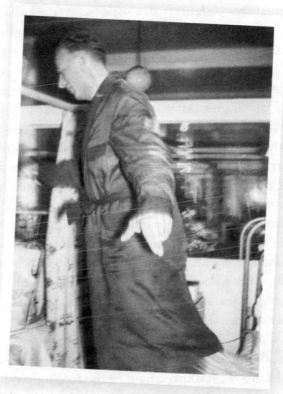

Jumping from bed to bed.

and looking after bladder drainage. I was swiftly marked as competent at performing all these tasks on adults.

I found it so much easier to do these procedures on an adult as they could understand why I was doing them and it was much easier to communicate with them. They weren't as small and delicate as children either, even though they occasionally behaved in the same way.

As well as learning to cope with the men's high jinks, I did learn some new things as well. It was here that I began to learn to care for patients with anuria (when the kidneys can't make urine). These patients were given a form of dialysis, in which a catheter is inserted into their abdominal cavity with a line hung on a drip stand. Cleansing fluid would be dripped into the patient and left for a period of time, then drained to remove waste products and toxins from their body, which is what their urine would have done. Once again, I was using my aseptic skills to prevent infection.

I was also given the opportunity to nurse a patient on a Bird respirator. This is a small, portable machine on a stand and is a positive pressure breathing device. It helped patients to breathe by blowing air into their lungs; they then breathed out when the pressure from the respirator was relaxed.

I was sorry when my time here ended; not only had it been hugely rewarding, but it had been a dynamic and welcome change of pace.

My second placement was on the male genito-urinary surgical ward, which specialised in the reproductive system and the urinary system. I was somewhat apprehensive about working here – men are very different to children, I was discovering. However, I was keenly aware of the pioneering work being carried out on that ward, which was also linked to the kidney and transplant unit.

I was to be involved in the pre- and post-operative nursing care of patients having prostatectomies (removal of the prostate gland), nephrectomies (removal of the kidneys), cystopic (bladder) examination, cystodiathermy (the removal of unwanted tissue from the bladder), ureterolithotomy (a removal of a stone from the bladder), and kidney transplants. I would also learn to care for patients having haemodialysis, the procedure that Hammersmith Hospital had been famous for pioneering. I observed the machine while it took blood from a patient's body and passed it through a filter to remove the toxins. It was a truly life-saving treatment.

During my time on this ward, Carol, my friend from school, got back in touch. She was now working in a solicitor's office in London. To me, this was the height of sophistication, quite a different world to mine.

"We must get together! How do you fancy a night out on Saturday night?" she asked.

"Great! Saturday is my day off! I would love to!" I replied.

"I thought we might go to the Hammersmith Palais and dance to Joe Loss and his Orchestra."

Joe Loss was the resident band leader at the Palais in the 1950s and early 1960s and living locally. I'd heard a lot about him.

"You know, I've never been to the Hammersmith Palais," I told Carol.

"And you've lived round here all these years. You don't know what you're missing. Ask the others." She insisted, "I'll pick you up in Dad's car."

"I think there could be quite a few of us off duty on Saturday night."

"The more the merrier!" she said. "It's Dad's huge Austin Cambridge estate so you can all squeeze in."

"Don't tell me your dad trusts you with his precious car?" I teased her.

"He does actually, but you know him – he's charging me sixpence a mile for the privilege!"

We laughed. I could just picture him.

"I'm not surprised," I said.

She turned up at our house in Putney as arranged and beeped the horn.

"Come on, everyone! Carol's here!" I herded my housemates together and we piled out of the house in our glad rags, excited at the prospect of a great evening ahead.

"Gosh!" Carol exclaimed when she saw me. "I've never seen you with short hair."

I gave a twirl and introduced her to the other girls.

"Vanessa looks so different," Carol said to my housemates. "I've only ever known her with plaits!"

We then packed ourselves into the huge estate, scrunched up together, and Carol drove off.

I remember having a great evening, going mad and doing the twist all together on the beautiful maple dance floor – not that you could see it in the crowd of so many pairs of feet. The music was fabulous, and Joe Loss was a brilliant band leader. We didn't know at the time that he would later be a patient at Hammersmith Hospital and, according to a student nurse who treated him, for all his fame he was always kind and gentlemanly to the nursing staff.[29]

Back on the ward, I had the opportunity to work in the separate sterile unit where patients were reverse barrier nursed following kidney transplants. In the early 1960s, the first immunosuppression drug was introduced. This was a drug aimed at preventing the body from rejecting the implant, but it also reduced the body's ability to fight infection (called immunosuppression). These patients were not only immunosuppressed, but had also undergone major surgery, so our reverse barrier nursing technique on this unit was even more rigorous than at GOS.

The cubicle couldn't be accessed directly. We covered our uniforms and shoes with a gown and special overshoes in an anteroom. If our hair wasn't short, we wore a head covering. Otherwise, the washing of hands on entering and leaving this sterile unit and the wearing and disposal of masks was the same as our reverse barrier nursing at GOS.

All sterile equipment and food for the patient was passed through a double hatch. The cubicle had its own crockery and cutlery. Nothing went through the hatch if it might be contaminated. The nurse caring for the patient would be specialling, so staff stayed with the patient until they were relieved by another member of staff at the end of the shift. On leaving the cubicle area, all outer uniform coverings were disposed of. Visitors waved at the patient through a glass partition.

As you might expect, there was a lot of urine involved on the genito-urinary surgical ward. One of our tasks was to do the "bottle round". We'd collect all the bottles of urine and put them into crates to carry to the sluice, where some poor first year would have the job of washing and sterilising them. The problem for us was that the men would do their very best to fill their bottles to the brim, so we struggled to lift them out of the bed holder without a spillage. We got through plenty of gloves and at times it didn't feel as though I'd had much of a promotion from the sluice.

But life was never boring. One day there was a fire drill. We usually knew the day these would take place, but never the time, so you couldn't prepare for it. When the alarm went, we had to act fast, as if it were for real. This meant evacuating the ward in record time, pushing all the patients in their beds to the designated area on the other side of the hospital. On this particular day I was running with another nurse as if we were in some kind of bizarre obstacle course. We had a full bottle of urine in a holder attached to the bed and the contents of the bottle were slopping all over my shoes.

"Put your back into it, Nurse," the patient joked.

I should've reprimanded him and told him how disgusting it was to fill the bottle so full, but I couldn't help but laugh.

As I was coming to the end of my stint on this ward, another situation forced me to think on the spot.

"Nurse, I'd like you to assist with the transfer of a surgical patient back to his psychiatric hospital."

Sister went on to explain who the patient was and briefed me on his background. I was more than happy to go on an outing. I'd be perfectly safe with the two ambulance crew members. Both of them would sit in the cab, one driving, the other ringing the bell as there were no sirens back then. However that day, as this journey was a non-emergency, they wouldn't need a bell.

"Hop in the back, Nurse," one of the crew said. "There's your seat, near the cab window so you can talk to us if there's any problem."

The patient sat compliantly in his seat and seemed calm enough. What could go wrong?

As it turned out, plenty. He might've been calm enough to start with, but once we'd been driving for five minutes or so, he suddenly leapt up and, before I had the chance to respond, he'd opened the rear doors of the ambulance and started swinging out over the road on one of them. We were travelling through London so weren't going very fast, but even so, it was very worrying. What if he let go?

I made a snap decision.

"I'm going to ignore the patient," I informed the crew.

They could see what was going on and would probably have stopped the ambulance or started ringing the bell, but because I assured them I had the situation in hand (I really didn't know for sure if I had), they carried on with the journey. Surely he wouldn't jump out at that speed, would he? Surely he was doing this for attention, wasn't he? Luckily, I was right. When he realised he was being ignored, he closed the doors and sat back down, meek as anything. The crew gave me a subtle thumbs up and I knew a crisis had been averted, whether through luck or judgement I'll never know. We had no further trouble from him.

On the way back to Hammersmith Hospital, I was squashed in the front with the crew and we were chatting. They were concerned about "the trauma I had suffered".

"I'm fine," I told them. "I'm more concerned about this rush hour traffic. I'm already late off duty and was hoping to get a lift home." Maggie sometimes had her father's car, and this was one time when she had brought it to the hospital.

"Right," the driver said, nodding at his mate. "This calls for action."

With that, the other crew member rang the bell, parting the traffic so that we returned in record time. I suspect this was illegal, and certainly today you can't sound a siren without authorisation from ambulance control. The nice thing was that Maggie had waited for me, which was a relief after the day's adventure.

My first introduction to night duty was on the gynae ward, which was run by a staff nurse who looked after me well. I did the pre- and post-operative care of patients admitted for various operations for women's health, hysterectomies (removal of the womb) and what we would call a D and C (usually removal of contents left in the womb) and an AP resection (removal of the rectum – lower part of your large bowel – for cancer). I was signed off as being competent to care for all these in my cross-chart booklet.

What I found interesting on this ward was that the women seemed to be far more demanding than the men I'd nursed at Hammersmith Hospital. When the women wanted their water jug refilled, they wanted it done there and then. They reminded me every time I was in the vicinity, even if I was rushing with a dressings trolley to pack a bleeding wound. The men, on the other hand, were much more patient. When I returned with a full jug of water, apologising for taking so long, they would say, "No bother, Nurse. I could see you were busy."

My second ward on night duty was D2, a mixed general surgical ward. I was told I would take charge there. The management at the Hammersmith trusted and respected our GOS training and they were giving us more and more responsibility. This ward was a huge step up for me. Today, some of the patients we looked after on this ward would be sent to an Intensive Care Unit. Thankfully there was support if I needed it. I had a night sister who assisted me regularly on the drug round and, although there were no bleeps at that time, the telephone switchboard were very prompt at finding me the appropriate person to come to my aid if I needed them.

This ward cared for patients following heart surgery. According to my cross-chart, I nursed patients having heart valve replacements, widening of the heart valves, and the closure of an opening in the heart (patients who would have had a hole in the heart as babies). All these patients would be nursed in a specialist coronary care unit today.

I remember these patients having drains in their wound that led to a bag that collected any excess blood. I had to measure this blood carefully and give the patient the exact amount of blood through their infusion to replace what was lost. This wasn't something one would ever do for children, as everything was written down on a prescription and calculated according to the child's weight. I was marked as competent to nurse other surgical patients as well, such as those following a mastectomy (removal of one or both breasts) and removal of both the thyroid gland and the gall bladder.

Another operation that was performed on more than one patient while I was on the ward was an operation to cut the connections to and from the frontal lobe of the brain, known as a frontal lobotomy. It was carried out in those days for the treatment of certain psychiatric conditions such as schizophrenia, depression and compulsive disorders. An article published in the BBC News magazine reports that it was a five-minute operation, very quickly done, but patients were never followed up properly. Decades later, an eminent neurosurgeon who followed up several 100 of these patients, commented that although patients *seemed* all right, they were totally ruined as social human beings. The operation rapidly fell out of favour, partly because of poor results but also because of the introduction of effective psychiatric medicines.[30]

I always worried about how these patients would react to this kind of surgery, but never had a problem with them after surgery as they were well sedated.

This ward was incredibly busy, but I had Hammersmith students who worked very hard to support me. We even had a patient on a ventilator in a side ward for a few nights who, because he was an adult, wasn't specialled. I remember that he was washed in the mornings and made comfortable by two of the Hammersmith students. When he was taken off the ventilator, he recalled to me a conversation that the students had had over his bed about their boyfriends. When I told the students about this, they were appalled.

"But we thought he was unconscious!" one of them exclaimed, slightly horrified.

"I suppose that's a lesson learned for all of us," I replied. "Never assume a patient in a coma can't hear you."

I didn't blame the nurses for chatting while they thought the patient couldn't hear them because there was hardly ever time for a break. This was probably just as well. Sitting on our chairs was never an option because of the minor inconvenience of the cockroaches.

The ward was in one of the old blocks due to be upgraded. It was direly needed. Cockroaches were a common infestation in old buildings, such as hospitals in London in the 1960s, and according to the internet still can be. Being nocturnal insects, they were attracted to the light from our lamp in the sitting area, which was why we didn't mind missing our breaks. We really didn't want to see the cockroaches scuttling around us. Crunching them underfoot was bad enough. Thankfully I never saw any cockroaches near a patient.

Sometimes when I returned home after my night shift, I worried that I hadn't cared for all my patients as well as I would have wanted. I remember one night having an elderly lady in one of our side rooms who was due to have an operation the following day. I'd helped her settle for the night and given her a bell to call me if she wanted anything. I had no chance to return to see how she was until early the following morning when her premedication was due.

"Did you manage to sleep?" I asked her.

She looked somewhat sheepish. Then she said, "I have a confession to make."

"Oh?" I said. "Is everything alright?"

"Well, it is now," she replied.

And then she explained what had happened. She'd wanted to go to the toilet in the middle of the night.

"But you were so busy," she said. "I didn't want to call you."

I wondered what on earth she was going to say.

"I know I shouldn't have," she said, looking concerned, "but I pulled my chair over to the sink and stood on it." There was a moment's pause when I realised what she was going to tell me. "I went to the toilet in the sink."

I was horrified. "We're *never* too busy to take you to the toilet," I told her.

"I did my best to clean the sink afterwards," she said.

"That's not what I'm worried about. You could so easily have fallen."

For the rest of the shift and many times since, I've wondered how this lady managed to perform such acrobatics. Although the chair in her room was a sturdy one, I wouldn't have dared to attempt what she did.

During my last week on this ward, I was about to go into the office to give the handover report to the day staff. The Hammersmith students were distributing the patients' breakfast.

"Please wake up, Mr Turner," one kept saying. "You need to eat your breakfast."

I went over to see if something was wrong. The patient wasn't responding. I could immediately see that he'd had a heart attack.

"Quickly, call the crash team," I said to her.

The student, previously unsure what to do, now leapt into action and rushed off. Mr. Turner was a substantial man. I needed to get him on to a hard surface. Somehow I got him off the bed and onto the floor on my own. To this day I'm not sure how I did it, but presumably my adrenaline kicked in and gave me the strength.

I was in the middle of performing external cardiac massage when the crash team arrived. I was relieved as this was exhausting work, much harder than it looks on television, but I was confused to notice that they weren't relieving me. They'd obviously spent a few moments watching me as I was surprised to feel one of the medical staff tucking the straps of my apron (which should have been pinned in place in a cross behind my back) into my waistband.

"Keep going, Nurse," he said. "You're doing a grand job!"

They didn't test my resilience for long. They took over very quickly, for which I was grateful. I must have looked very dishevelled though!

On another occasion, a staff nurse from the ward went home with the keys to the medicines trolley and cupboards – a mortal sin, and something for which we would undoubtedly have been disciplined at GOS. I was left a telephone message to say the keys were on their way back to me. I hoped they'd hurry up as we were stuck without them.

Suddenly, a policeman came onto the ward asking for me: "Nurse Owen?"

"Yes, Officer. May I help you?"

"I've got something to give you." He handed over an envelope bearing my name.

"Gosh, are these our drug keys?" I could see from the bulging envelope that the keys were inside. "Thank you so much, Officer. You're a lifesaver."

I thanked him profusely, and he was charming, saying that he was delighted to help. But I was shocked. How did the staff nurse have the confidence to walk into her local station and ask the police to do this?

CHANGE ON THE HORIZON

Most Sundays throughout my childhood, I attended an Anglican Church in Barnes with my mother. Now, working in hospital and particularly working shifts, I had very few Sundays free. Even if I did, I was often too exhausted to make the journey home to attend church.

The priest began to remonstrate with me. "I know you're now working in a hospital but I do expect you to attend church more regularly," he told me one Sunday after the service.

"I'm exhausted," I told him. "I've just come off a run of 12-hour night shifts."

"I'm sure you can be more organised," he told me. "I would like to see you make more of an effort."

I was at home for my four nights off duty and thought about what this vicar had said. He couldn't have made me feel less welcome. I knew some people who attended a church in East Sheen so I enquired about the services there. There appeared to be many more to choose from.

"Why not come to evensong at 6.30 p.m. and then to our youth club afterwards," one of my neighbours suggested. "You'd be made very welcome."

I began to attend Christ Church in East Sheen. It had a larger congregation than my church in Barnes with a number of young people attending. It was lovely for church to be a relaxing respite after a long run of shifts, rather than a cause for even more stress.

It was at one of these youth club meetings after church that I met a young curate. He'd recently been made a deacon, arriving in the parish only six weeks before. At this particular meeting, there was music playing and a lot of us were dancing in a group to the music. This curate was persuaded to join us. I immediately noticed his utter lack of rhythm. Although I didn't think much about the meeting, I later found out he'd enquired and learnt from a fellow curate that I was a student nurse working in a hospital not too far away.

When he had his three-week summer holiday, he spent the first week trying to find me. He didn't have much to go on other than my name and occupation, but he persisted. He toured around hospitals just north of the Thames and west of London, asking to see the matron to ask if she had a Nurse Owen on her staff. He remembers that Chelsea and Westminster Hospital had a male matron, unusual for the 1960s, who exclaimed, "Oh, you young men!"

I received a note in my pigeonhole from the matron at Hammersmith Hospital. On one side it had his name and phone number and on the other a note from Matron herself.

"This young man called to see you. Should you wish to contact him, his number is on the reverse."

I could imagine the tone of her voice as I read it. Who was this young man? Then I remembered: The youth club. The dancing. The curate with no rhythm! *Should I call him? He'd gone to all this trouble to find me. He must be planning something in the parish and he wants me to be involved.*

I phoned his number that afternoon. I didn't realise it, but I was phoning his parents' home number.

"Is John Martin there?"

"Is that Vanessa? Can we meet?"

"Yes, I'm sure we can."

"Can you meet me tonight?"

"That might be a bit difficult."

He laughed. I remembered he had quite an embarrassing laugh.

I thought about it briefly. I had the night off, but I'd already arranged to meet up with my old school friend Carol. Typical, I thought. I hardly ever had the time or energy to go out and now I was double-booked. Carol was meeting her boyfriend, Ralf. He was travelling down to London with a Scottish rugby team.

"The problem is that I'm meeting an old friend and her boyfriend in a pub tonight."

"Oh." He sounded disappointed. There was a pause. "Could I disturb you there?"

"Her boyfriend's on tour with his rugby team," I told him.

"I think I could cope with that."

I could hear the smile in his voice. I had nothing to lose. "All right then, I'm sure Carol won't mind."

When I arrived at the pub, I found Carol surrounded by a pack of rugby players. She seemed quite happy. I was looking forward to catching up with her because she was living in Scotland and we hardly saw one another, but I was curious about why this keen young curate wanted to see me.

"Vanessa!"

Carol shouted when she spotted me, "Come here, let me introduce you."

She did indeed introduce me to the whole rugby team

while I smiled awkwardly and greeted the team of uninhibited Scotsmen. Then John arrived. He bought me a drink and we chatted, though it was hard to hear above the noise.

"Shall we go for a meal?" he said after 20 minutes or so.

"I've eaten," I said.

"I'm starving," he said. "Would you come along with me anyway?"

"I'm not sure. I've hardly spoken to Carol and I don't like to abandon her." Then I looked at Carol, who was having a whale of a time surrounded by all those men. "I don't see why not."

We found a Chinese restaurant close by the pub. It was small, not too busy and lovely and quiet.

We ordered a meal and I managed to eat a little. It was sometime later that his mother told me that John had had a very good supper that night already.

I found it easy to talk to John. He certainly asked me about my family.

Over a pudding of lychees, his favourite, he told me about his background.

"My parents met in the Sudan," he said. "They were CMS missionaries."

"CMS?"

"Church Mission Society. My mother was a teacher there, the deputy head of the first-ever Sudanese girls' school at Omdurman."

"And your father?"

"He was running a mission station at Salara, a village in the Nuba Mountains where there was a mud church, a primary school and a dispensary."

"Was this during the war?"

"Yes, they married in 1940 in Khartoum Cathedral and lived in the mission station bungalow. Dad had tried to enlist as a chaplain in the army, but after the third attempt he was told he would be imprisoned if he tried again. The authorities felt that his role should be a reserved occupation. He was needed where he was."

"Were you born here in Britain?"

"No, my younger brother and I were both born in Khartoum Hospital."

"Gosh, can you remember anything about it?"

"It was certainly different. Salara, my first home, was a Stone Age village of mud huts where no one wore clothes, apart from the married women who wore beads around their waists. The tribal chief had a pink lady's corset, which he wore on ceremonial occasions."

"Where on earth had he got that from?"

"We never found out. The Nubas were fascinated that Dad had two pairs of shorts. They asked him why, if he was so wealthy, he didn't display them by wearing both at once. They would have. My mother was told by the villagers that she was worth 15 piasters. It was intended to be a complement. It was a high price for a wife and worth about three shillings in those days in the Nuba Mountains."

"Presumably the Nubas had very little money?"

"A Nuba would earn a piaster for a day's work during the war."

"Can you remember any of this?"

"I have some memories. We lived on the other side of a dirt road from the village until I was three and a half. I remember swallows nesting on the veranda and the little .410 shotgun that we kept for killing snakes. I thought the gun was seven feet tall, but I must have been very young then. Then the war ended, and we came back to Britain. Everything looked and felt and sounded different. Dad's a vicar in Surbiton now. That's where I'm staying for the rest of my holiday."

"Surbiton must feel a far cry from Africa," I mused. "What a life you've lived."

"I don't work in a hospital like you," he said. "You must have had experiences of your own."

"I suppose I have," I said.

"In that case, how about we go out again tomorrow and you can tell me all about them?"

"Yes, all right," I said. "Why not?"

John still had two weeks left. He arranged to see me on the next couple of evenings before I went back on night duty.

"How long do you need to sleep during the day after your nights?" he asked me on the second evening.

"That depends . . ."

"Is it possible to see you in the afternoon before you go on duty?"

"I don't see why not."

We arranged that he'd pick me up at three o'clock the next day. I set an alarm and asked a housemate to double-check I was awake because I needed time to get ready.

We went for a walk and had a picnic. He remembered me mentioning I liked lemon meringue pie and brought a whole one!

"Gosh," I said. "I don't think I can eat a whole pie."

"How about half?" he joked. "I'm rather partial to lemon meringue too."

Over the next two weeks, he'd collect me and my housemates every morning when we came off duty. We'd all squeeze into his father's little Ford car and he'd drive us home. It was much quicker than catching the bus. My housemates were thrilled.

Not put off by my housemates, John proposed to me at the end of his holiday. Later, he told me it took him only three days from our first meeting to decide that he wanted to marry me and a further 10 days to pluck up the courage to ask. It took me double that to decide to accept his proposal!

Back on day duty, I spent another six weeks on an orthopaedic ward. I remember little about this ward, except learning how to set up traction on a patient's leg as he had a broken thigh bone. A frame was set up around the bed, with a series of weights, ropes and pulleys to exert force on his leg and keep the bone in the correct position during the early stages of healing. I also learnt how to apply a Denis Browne splint, used for the treatment of a deformity of the foot, and how to apply plaster of Paris to a limb. I was signed as competent to look after patients following a meniscectomy (the removal of damaged cartilage in the knee joint) and also for an amputation of the lower leg. This required giving the patient both physical and emotional support.

While I was working on this ward, I developed laryngitis. I couldn't speak. I didn't feel especially unwell, nor did I have a temperature, so the sister suggested I did paperwork in the office. It was very strange just to be sitting down and not rushing around the ward, so strange in fact that another member of staff took this photo of me. "Shirker," she joked. Although I laughed, not much sound came out.

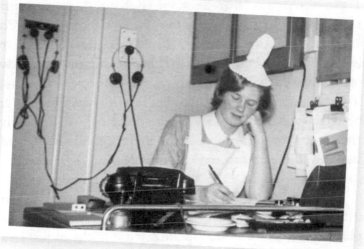

Me with laryngitis.

Finally the six of us spent our last three months at Hammersmith Hospital in the obstetrics unit, where we were to do formal training in pregnancy and childbirth. Here we had our first formal lectures. Another excellent sister tutor was responsible for our experience and teaching. We had to observe a specific number of deliveries (normal, breech and forceps, as well as caesarean sections) and we had to care for the mothers. As staff knew we were from GOS, they were confident that we needed no instruction in bathing newborn babies and performing their birth examination to make sure they had no obvious physical problems. They realised that this task wasn't a challenge for us as we'd been surrounded by babies in our first two years. The Hammersmith midwives took advantage of this and frequently relied on our help when they were busy.

There were many links between GOS and Hammersmith Hospital, one being that they both had royal patronage. The relationship between the two hospitals was encouraged by Professor Moncrieff, who had a special interest in diseases of the newborn baby. He instigated the opening of the first-ever neonatal intensive care unit with eight cots in the obstetrics department at Hammersmith Hospital. He'd been giving lectures and demonstrations to postgraduate medical students in the unit from December 1947.

It was during the 1950s that GOS nursing students began to be seconded to this baby unit. My friend Patricia, who you may remember mistook a consultant physician for a plumber in her first year, spent three months of her final year of training in this unit. Patricia remembers how she was regularly singled out to assist a paediatric registrar in performing exchange transfusions of newborn babies with jaundice. This is when a baby's blood is removed and exchanged with donor blood. It's a lifesaving procedure and was pioneering work at that time.

Working on this unit reminded Patricia of when her father, a respected consultant surgeon who treated adults, once visited her while she was working with newborn babies at GOS. He had experience of treating troops on the front line and was contemptuous of her wanting to train as a children's nurse, believing it was just a form of "nannying". During his visit, he was able to watch her at work and was astounded by the responsibilities that the GOS nurses had for very sick babies. He was overwhelmed by their expertise. She never forgot how his attitude to her career choice changed totally after that visit. It was the recognition of

GOS nurses' professionalism that contributed, I believe, to the responsibility we were given at Hammersmith Hospital.

At the end of our three months on the obstetrics unit, we had to sit an examination and then have a viva (an oral exam). During this, we were warned that a consultant obstetrician would fire random questions at us relating to our training. They expected prompt answers. Because this was something we had never experienced before, we found the prospect quite stressful to say the least. When it was my turn, I had a number of questions fired at me in quick succession. I remember that the final one was about the signs and symptoms of pre-eclampsia. I was so glad that I knew the answer and was able to respond immediately.

"A high blood pressure, swelling of the ankles and the presence of protein in the urine," I replied straight away.

But this wasn't all. He questioned me further. "And can you tell me how it is treated, Nurse?"

"Yes, if possible, by inducing the birth of the baby but primarily by admission to hospital for careful observation and bed rest."

I really hoped I'd done enough to pass.

Thankfully I had.

At the end of this obstetrics course we were given a certificate which, if we wanted to go on to train to be a midwife, would shorten the course by three months. Then there were two further hurdles to negotiate – one a written exam, the other a practical exam taken by an outside examiner – before we became state registered nurses.

I remember feeling very confident about the practical exam. We were given scenarios for which we had to prepare a patient and treat them appropriately. It always included setting up a trolley to test our procedure using an aseptic technique, which I was something of an expert in after my six weeks in the GOS theatres. When these exams were completed (and luckily all passed), this part of our training was over. At last, we were able to return to GOS, not only as fourth-year sick children's students, but also as qualified adult-trained nurses.

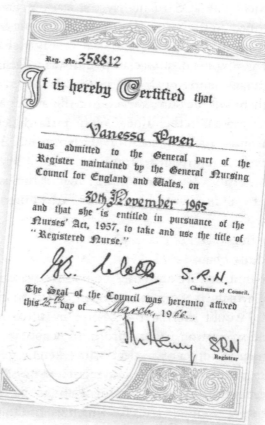

General Nursing Council Certificate.

FOURTH YEAR: GOS

Our fourth year at GOS seemed very strict compared with the much more relaxed atmosphere at the Hammersmith, but we had the advantage of a new-found confidence from working away. We had to leave our Putney residence, but we were allowed to live out in one of the authorised nurses' homes rather than the one attached to the hospital.

I was allocated a room in the Coram Street residence, an impressive building that was also warden controlled, though at this stage in our training the warden was protective to us, not restrictive. We had to buy our own gaberdine mac and hat to wear outside when it rained, but we were given wonderful long capes to wear when walking the short journey to the hospital.

This was our management year, and we were training to become staff nurses. We were expected to take responsibility for a children's ward at night, oversee more junior staff and take over the staff nurse's role when she was elsewhere. We also oversaw junior staff performing dressings, suture removal and assisting with medical procedures.

Our first few weeks were spent back in the nursing school, revising our care of sick children. Among other things, we were taught dietetics and artificial feeding by Dr Philip Evans, a consultant physician and director of child health. We also learned about cardiac surgery and diseases of the digestive tract from Mr David Waterston, consultant heart surgeon, and about tumours and the treatment of diseases of the brain by Mr George Macnab, consultant neurosurgeon.

I still lacked a lot of paediatric nursing experience so I was excited to discover that I'd been allocated Ward 1A, the cardiothoracic (heart) unit, which was the first of its kind in the world. This wing had been the vision and initiative of two highly respected and experienced doctors specialising in cardiology, Mr David Waterston (surgeon) and Dr Richard Bonham-Carter (a physician and medical practitioner who specialised in the diagnosis and treatment of heart conditions by other than surgical means. Interestingly he was a distant relation of Florence Nightingale). They wanted the research facilities and the diagnosis and treatment of paediatric heart disease under one roof. Both medical and surgical diseases of the chest were treated jointly in this unit. Although the building of this unit began in early 1960, it wasn't opened in its entirety until 1988 because of various complications.[31/32] I started working in the new part of the unit in November 1965.

The surgeons were famous for their pioneering surgery. We had many children flown not only from across the country but also from across the whole world to take advantage of these surgeons' and Dr Bonham-Carter's expertise. There was even an area in Coram's Fields next to the hospital, where we had a makeshift helipad. We put out a large white sheet to help the helicopter see where to land. Sick children could be flown to us for treatment in record time, even from other countries, which was unique in those days.

Working on 1A was exciting. I began by nursing a child with Fallot's tetralogy, commonly known as "blue baby syndrome". This condition affected the child's heart structure and function. The child I nursed had a temporary operation before he was old enough to have his complete repair, designed to improve how much oxygen was in the blood circulating around his body. I also cared for a child on a Bird respirator, the small machine on a stand to help with breathing (which I had used at Hammersmith Hospital).

The experience I remember most was caring for two children with transposition of the great arteries, where the arteries leaving the heart were the wrong way round. This means that the blood from the lungs (containing oxygen) flows back to the lungs, and the blood to the heart (which has given up its oxygen to the body) flows back to the body. It was, and remains, one of the most challenging forms of heart disease to treat. One in 5,000 babies is born with this condition.[33] Children born with this condition are also referred to as blue babies. They often die at birth but, if they survive, it's often because they have a hole in the heart. As soon as they're diagnosed, they need emergency surgery to allow more mixing of the blue and the red blood so that some oxygen is able to get around their body.

One child I cared for was a young boy, Edward, who was five and a half. Edward had what we call a shunt; an emergency operation to create a passage connecting the two main arteries of his heart. This was performed by Mr Waterston when Edward was only six weeks old.

Edward was now in hospital for his full repair. He was to have this repair performed by Mr Eoin Aberdeen, a consultant since 1963, who was renowned for an impressive series of Mustard operations for the treatment of transposition of the great arteries.[34] Mr Aberdeen performed more of these operations than any other surgeon in the UK. The pioneer was Dr William Mustard, who in 1963 had first transposed the great arteries in a Toronto hospital using a heart and lung bypass machine.[35]

It was a very new operation at the time. It was now 1965, and Edward's was to be the twenty-third repair carried out by Mr Aberdeen. Because operating on a beating heart is extremely difficult, the bypass machine would take over the role of the heart and lungs. It had taken five years until the first-ever children's heart and lung bypass machine was ready to use at GOS, following painstaking design and testing in the unit's research department. The first operation using this machine was performed in 1962, the year I started my training.[35]

Edward was a lovely boy whose care I was allowed to take over now I was in my fourth year. It was during the week before Christmas that I prepared him for theatre for his Mustard operation. Following the repair and his disconnection from the bypass machine, I was to assist with his care in the two bedded "pump room", where there was more space, for the first few days. Then I would take over specialling him. He had a temporary tracheostomy, which by now I was very confident to look after, and he was on an Engström ventilator, which took over his breathing entirely.

Great Ormond Street's Engström ventilators were the cutting-edge technology of the day. They were so large that, with an oxygen cylinder, they took up a quarter of a side room. If a child in the hospital needed the care that an intensive care nurse would give today, the equipment (as well as the registered nurse) went to the speciality ward itself and the child was "specialled". (These days, the child would leave their ward and be taken to a paediatric intensive care unit (PICU).) The Engström ventilators were set up by an anaesthetist who monitored them regularly. They were maintained and sometimes even rebuilt by Dr Graham, a physiologist based on 1A.

I needed to learn how to monitor and regularly record the readings from this ventilator. Edward also had underwater seal drainage, where a tube from his chest would drain any blood, fluid or air that had collected around the lungs during surgery, through a sealed bottle of sterile water. I had learnt to look after these at Hammersmith Hospital.

Edward's parents, Pat and George, visited him daily, travelling on the Underground from Loughton. I got to know them very well and Pat still keeps in contact with me to this day, 56 years later. Edward had an older sister, Kay, who was 10, and a brother, Alan, just under a year older, at six and a half. Alan, who I am still in touch with and have had many calls and emails with, tells me:

"There were five weeks each year when Edward and I were the same age. The only thing was, I minded a bit having to go to bed at the same time as Edward for those five weeks. For the rest of the year I was allowed to stay up for an extra 15 minutes!"

Once Edward had been taken off the ventilator, Pat and George were allowed to bring Edward's siblings to 1A to reassure them that he was OK. This would have been two or three days after the operation.

Alan recalls: "I had been told that Edward was fine. I was too small to see through the round window of the pump room door, so I had to be lifted up to see my brother. The bed was facing the door. Edward was sitting propped up on a pillow with tubes all over him. Bunny was propped up on the pillow beside him. (Bunny was his favourite toy.) I could see that he was OK because Bunny was with him and he wasn't blue anymore. I remember it as a nice experience."

Pat told me about Bunny. He had been knitted by her elderly nanny when Edward was born. Edward had never been parted from him. "Each evening when we had to leave Edward, we told him, 'we have to go now but we'd see you tomorrow.' Edward would hug Bunny to him as if he was saying, 'Bunny will look after me now.'"

There were no facilities for parents to stay at that time, so Pat and George stayed the night after Edward's operation in a hotel near to the hospital so that they could be nearby. Once they knew he was quite safe and recovering, they went back to visiting him daily. The hospital had no eating and rest facilities for parents either, but apparently they were able to eat in a café around the corner from the hospital. This gave them a break and some fresh air, as the hospital was very hot.

I was on 1A for Christmas, my third Christmas spent at GOS. This year I did manage to get to the doctors' revue in the nurses' home dining room, which I appreciated more than usual as I knew many of the doctors that the songs and sketches were about. I remember a song about Mr James Crooks, the ENT consultant with whom I'd worked. It was about him not liking any noise in theatre while he operated. There was a regular "shush, shush" and "Jim, Jim" in the song and a line about "Stop the clock ticking". The audience were beside themselves. I appreciated it as I remembered being lectured about having a good breakfast before my spell with him in theatre, well aware he wouldn't appreciate it if one of us had made a noise by fainting.

1A was decorated and the windows painted. Alan remembers that the theme was Winnie-the-Pooh and that his and Edward's Uncle Joe helped with the painting as he was a talented artist. On Christmas and Boxing Day, even with double the staff, 1A was still busier than the other wards where I'd spent previous Christmases. A rota was drawn up by one of the sisters so that we each spent a regular two hours responsible for a child or children we knew well (one of mine being Edward). This was followed by a two-hour break in the cosy corner so we could chat and enjoy our Christmas dinner and the various chocolates given by parents.

By now, Edward was off his ventilator, his temporary tracheostomy had been closed, and his chest drain removed. He'd been moved from the pump room into the four-bedded ward and was only having his oxygen tent at night if he needed it. In the daytime he was up and about and gradually regaining his strength.

We had dressing-up clothes on the ward and the children who were able to get out of bed wore costumes. One of the staff picked out costumes for Edward. He was getting stronger and cheekier every day. I can tell that Edward's hand is holding my arm in the photograph because I'm wearing my engagement ring – a sin on any other day of the year.

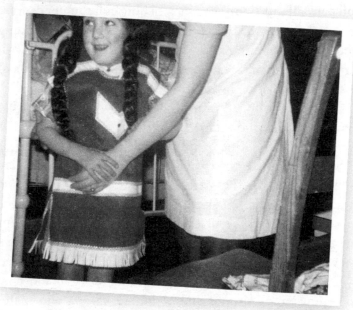

Edward dressed up at Christmas.

Of course, Father Christmas came around on Christmas morning. In the afternoon, the BBC broadcast its regular Christmas programme from the hospital. This year we had the comedian Frankie Howerd as the presenter instead of Max Bygraves. He was quite a different character from Max. He was loud, and made a lot of gestures. The news came back to the wards that some children were actually frightened of him. We understood that a plea went around the hospital for older, more confident children to be brought down from the wards, hoping they'd be happy to be interviewed. I'm not sure if the broadcast that year was as successful as previous years.

Edward's parents came to visit on Christmas afternoon with Alan, his sister Kay and Pat and George's godson, Michael. Alan came dressed as a policeman, much to the

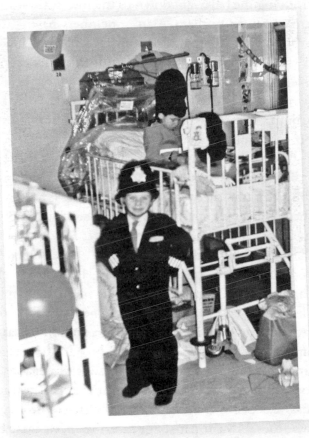

Edward's brother Alan and Edward on Christmas Day. Alan in his policeman outfit. Edward in the bed behind him in his guard's uniform (his oxygen tent is rolled away behind the pillow).

amusement of his brother. Pat doesn't remember a lot about that day. Alan, though, remembers Michael having a very bouncy ball for Christmas, as this was all the rage at the time. He remembers Michael, his mum and him climbing the hospital stairs to the top floor, leaning over the balustrade and dropping the ball right down to the lowest floor trying to get it to return to them. Alan remembers having to retrieve the ball a number of times from the floors below, but thinks that it did return to the seventh floor occasionally. He also remembers them going to an area where there was a huge rocking horse to ride. I expect this was the playroom by the outpatient department where children from 1A were taken occasionally for an outing.

On Boxing Day, I was able to remove the stitches from Edward's wound, which was another step in his recovery. Not long after that he was able to go home. Edward lived until he was an adult, married and had a daughter. Sadly, he died at the age of 30. His daughter still has Edward's Bunny. She had a son of her own on 1 August 2019 and named him Isaac Edward, a great-grandson for Pat. He's a lovely child and I have a picture of him on my living room mantlepiece. Pat asked me to add that she always remembers Edward as a 30-year-old and now imagines him as a young 30-year-old grandfather.

During my time spent on 1A, John was still a deacon. He had to have permission from his bishop to marry during this first year of his training. He was in lodgings, so a flat had to be found by the parish for us to live in. He was being ordained as a priest in June 1966 and was given permission to marry in the July. I then had to negotiate with Gwen Kirby, our matron, as to whether I would be allowed to marry as I wouldn't finish my nurse training until the end of September that year. At that time, I knew of no student who'd been allowed to get married before they qualified. I gather now that there was one other.

I made an appointment with Miss Kirby. As kind as she was, I was always a bit nervous when going to her office.

"Take a seat, Nurse," she said. "What can I do for you?"

"May I have your permission to get married?" I said, thinking I'd best get straight to it. After all, Matron's time was precious so there was no point pussyfooting around.

"Married. I see." There was a moment's pause. "Tell me a little about your fiancé."

It wasn't an out-and-out no, so that was something.

"His name is John. He's a curate in East Sheen parish at the moment. He's going to be ordained in June."

I told her about his missionary parents, his birth in the Sudan and how he had lived in the Nuba Mountains until he was three and a half.

"And where did John do his theological training?"

"King's College, London."

"Really?" Her face lit up. "I know the Dean, Canon Sidney Evans."

It was clear that Matron not only attended all the services in the hospital chapel but moved in the same circles as the Dean. She was relaxed, chatted a little more to me and I began to feel hopeful.

"I'll talk to the hospital board," she said. "And ask them if they would agree to your being married in July."

"Thank you very much, Matron," I said.

That was as far as she was able to make a commitment, but I knew I could trust her. When Gwendoline Kirby wanted something done, it usually got done. A good illustration of this was recounted by her niece, Sally Moyes. In 1950, when she first became matron at GOS, Miss Kirby was determined to find a way into the hospital's senior meetings.

"She commandeered the tea trolley, served drinks to the hospital's nursing committee and sat down and joined them," said Sally. "No one at the table dared to ask her to go away. From then on, she was included in all the meetings. She was good at getting what she wanted. She had attended every nursing committee from 1950 and every Hospital for Sick Children board of governors meeting from 1953, until her retirement in 1969."[36]

I didn't have long to wait. Matron contacted me following the board meeting to tell me that permission had been granted: I was getting married.

My next allocation was two-weeks experience in the milk kitchen helping with the preparation of the baby feeds that were regularly distributed around the hospital. The milk kitchen was designed to be infection-free, so we had to gown up, cover our hair with a cap and wear overshoes. I spent time preparing feeds for babies on special diets that had been prescribed by the dietitian. We would have special formulas for the medical wards where children with skin conditions and diarrhoea and vomiting were tried on different milk formulas, mostly excluding cows' milk. There were also expressed milk banks, which I later contributed to when I was breastfeeding my own children. This breast milk could be prescribed for children with severe allergies when their mother was unable to breast-feed them.

My next ward was 6A&B, where one half of the ward was orthopaedic (muscles, bones and joints) and the other half renal (kidney problems). I spent seven weeks here. Again I returned to nurse renal conditions but I also had experience of fractures (broken bones) and the application and care of plaster of Paris, this time on children. I learnt to apply skin traction for a broken thigh bone in a similar way to how they'd done it at Hammersmith Hospital. We attached wide pink Elastoplast to the sides of a child's lower leg. The Elastoplast attached to ropes and was reinforced with bandages. The ropes turned on pulleys with weights on their end. These aligned the broken bone and would keep it in the right position for healing to take place.

I remember one evening sitting at the nurses' station, writing what we called the Kardex, which contained the nursing records of the children on the ward. There happened to be three young boys in bed and on traction in this bay. Being confined to bed for a number of weeks wasn't very stimulating for three boys, even though a teacher visited them from the hospital school every weekday.

The conversations between the boys were often amusing, with one boy often trying to outdo the others by saying he was better at something than they were. This particular evening, we were getting ready for visiting time and the boys were waiting for their parents. They were all talking about their fathers. One of the boys started to brag about how far away his dad could stand and still manage to aim his wee into the toilet. The conversation began to escalate or deteriorate, depending on which way you want to look at it.

"My dad can reach the toilet standing at the toilet door."

"My dad can do it from *outside* the toilet door."

"Mine can do it from the top of the stairs!"

The next moment, the parents walked into the ward. I found it hard to keep a straight face. As I saw these dads greeting their sons, I wondered how they would have felt had they overheard that conversation – maybe embarrassed but probably not surprised.

My 13 weeks of night duty were spent on 5A&B, a general medical ward. As a fourth year, I was now in charge of this ward and supporting a second-year student with her management skills. We were overseen by a night sister who checked the children's medicines with me and was available for any emergencies.

As I have no record of my work on this ward in my cross-chart book, presumably I must have completed all my medical competencies by then. I do have a few labelled pictures of children from the ward confirming that 5A&B specialised in autoimmune conditions (when healthy tissue is destroyed by the body's own immune system).

I nursed a child with coeliac disease, which is when the immune system attacks the lining of a person's small bowel when they eat gluten. I also nursed a child with Still's disease, a rare arthritis and autoimmune disease in babies, in which there are too many white cells and too few red ones in the blood.

The ward had a number of babies and children under five. Having so many young children on the ward was challenging from early in the morning. It was expected that not only were all the babies to have their 6 a.m. feed before the day staff arrived at 7.30 a.m., but all the children were washed and dressed and the tables in the playroom were laid for breakfast. Your organisation and management skills

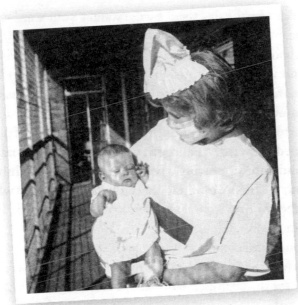

Me with a baby on the balcony in fourth year.

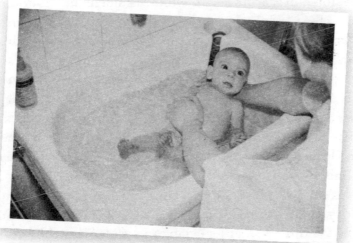

A baby in a cubicle sink.

were judged by the day sister by the state of your ward when she came on duty.

One morning, I appeared to have everything in pristine condition with all the children washed and dressed and the babies all fed. I'd even managed to lay the tables for breakfast early (at about 4 a.m.). Suddenly, at about 7.15, I noticed with horror a toddler standing in his cot in the corner of the ward. He'd somehow managed to remove his soiled nappy. Not only had he smeared the cot, himself (face and hair included) with poo, but he'd also plastered the nearby walls.

I called for my first-year student companion.

"How has he managed that?" she asked in disbelief. "He was all nice and clean a moment ago!"

"I have no idea," I said, taken aback myself, but there was no time for dithering. "He needs to go into the bath. Quick as you can!"

She hesitated just for a moment, then scooped him up, keeping him at arm's length, while rushing to the bathroom down the corridor. Meanwhile I had to dispose of the bed linen and scrub the cot and walls. Even the best-made plans don't always work out when you're a children's nurse.

We were just finishing the mammoth clear-up when we heard the sound of the lifts heralding the arrival of the day staff. I took some children into the playroom to sit them down at the tables ready for breakfast. Just as I thought I was finally ready to give the handover report, I heard a tinkling sound.

A child had already taken himself into the playroom. The windows there included a small pane at the bottom. It had a ring catch and opened on a slide. This child had collected all the cutlery from the tables and was having great fun posting each item one by one through the opened window and listening to the loud tinkling sound as they hit the concrete pavement five floors below.

I called for my first-year student. She came rushing in, having just cleaned up the toddler, and I handed her the five-year-old boy.

"Can you keep this one away from the cutlery while I make a phone call?"

She looked bemused but did as I had asked while I rushed to phone the front hall porter.

"He did what?" The hall porter laughed out loud. Once he'd recovered himself, he was very obliging. "I'll arrange for a hospital porter to collect the cutlery and return it to the ward."

"You're a lifesaver. Thank you so much."

As quick as anything, the cutlery was back in place and, thankfully, the ward sister, Sister Leavesley, was also amused by the early morning's mishaps and had been waiting patiently for my late handover report.

One thing emerged very clearly from all of these shenanigans. I vowed that if I ever became a sister running my own ward, I would always allow the night staff to let babies wake naturally for their 6 a.m. feed and I'd only expect children to be up, washed and dressed if they were awake and ready to get out of bed. In later years, I remembered my vow. It saved a lot of these last-minute panics.

A MARRIED STUDENT

John was priested in the June, but I missed the occasion as I was working my stretch of eight nights. I finished night duty at the beginning of July and we were married on the ninth. The wedding took place in Christ Church, East Sheen, one of the three churches where John was a curate and the church where I'd attended and joined the youth club.

Our wedding was taken by John's lovely father, and the best man was his younger brother. I had three bridesmaids: my little sister, Maria, who was now six years old; a young cousin of John's; and the daughter of good family friends who lived next door to my grandmother.

When I arrived at the church, I was shocked to find how full it was. As well as our family and friends, there were parishioners in the congregation from all three churches overflowing into the aisles. The choir stalls were full of choristers from all three churches; the younger members had to sit on the floor. A lady in a wheelchair had pride of place. I didn't know any of these people but was touched by the turnout.

Our organist was an exceptionally talented young man. He had perfect pitch. Even though John wasn't much of a singer, this chap could play the responses for the choir to sing in whichever key John happened to be singing.

I had complete faith when I asked him to play some challenging music – which included a Bach Fugue and Widor's Toccata in F. He didn't let us down. John still reminds me of how I "dug him in the ribs" during the first hymn. He says frequently, "She wouldn't even let me sing at my own wedding!" It seemed a shame to spoil the lovely music.

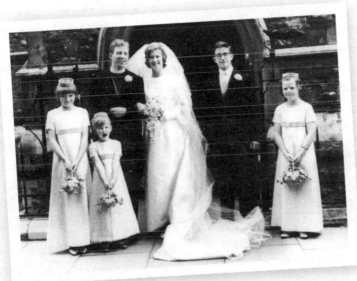

Our wedding– clearly a very tiring day for my little sister!

Our honeymoon was a week in a cottage lent to us by friends of John's parents, near Robin Hood's Bay in North Yorkshire. We hired the cheapest two-seater we could find. It was an olive-green BMC mini-van. When we arrived at the cottage, we found the only access was across a field. It had been raining and the van's little wheels got stuck in a rut. The only way we could move it was if I got behind and pushed while John tried to accelerate. I hadn't passed my driving test yet. We got the car moving, but I was covered in mud and my brand new pale yellow mac was completely ruined – not a good start to married life.

We decided to spend the week experiencing each other's hobbies. I took John riding. John, as a first-time rider, was given a horse that was far too docile. We spent our whole experience trying to stop his horse eating the hedges and the grass. I never even managed to get my horse to trot. Then John took me fly fishing. I found learning to cast a line almost impossible. I always got it tangled in a tree or a bush, from which, needless to say, he had to rescue it.

Then we spent another day painting with water-colours. John is a talented artist and always makes our Christmas cards. We sat on the beach, painting the headland of Robin Hood's Bay. John chose to paint one prominent house on the cliff and finished it speedily. I chose to paint a whole line of houses which took me ages. He had to hold an umbrella over my head while I tried to finish my painting in the rain.

It was over all too quickly and we returned to London. It had been a busy few weeks, with night duty and then preparations for the big day, but it was exciting to be venturing on this next journey in life. Both of us now had to carry on with our training.

On Monday 18 July I was back at GOS, ready to start my next training experience, six weeks working in the outpatient department (OPD). I spent my first three weeks in OPD experiencing different clinics, including general medical, surgical, orthopaedic and eyes. My role was to make sure that whichever clinic I had been allocated ran efficiently.

On the family's arrival I would collect the child's notes from reception and accompany them to see the consultant. I would sit in on the consultation and afterwards check that the family understood what they'd been told. It's easy to forget the details when you're emotionally involved in unfamiliar or even frightening circumstances. After this, if the child required further tests, I would take them to the appropriate department.

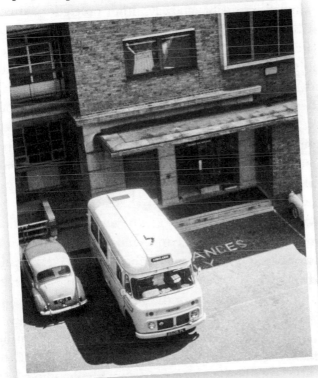

The outpatient entrance.

I also experienced how the hospital coped with families who arrived with a child in need of emergency care. Although there was no accident and emergency department at GOS, children were regularly referred from other paediatric units and brought to the hospital by ambulance. Local families would walk in off the street. The latter were never turned away. An area was set aside where a senior registrar would assess these children, then either treat or refer them to the appropriate speciality and arrange admission if necessary. Children with chronic illnesses, who were regular patients with us, had a card which they either brought to the unit or took to their GP. This enabled them to be transferred urgently by ambulance to us. They were then seen quickly and admitted to the appropriate ward, where they would already be known.

There was a large play area behind outpatients to occupy children while they were waiting for their appointment. I remember a baby born with a condition called oesophageal atresia being wheeled there in her buggy from Ward 1A. Her oesophagus – the tube that takes food from the throat to the stomach – had a blind end to it so there was no way this child could feed normally. The other end of her oesophagus, leading up from the stomach, was connected to her windpipe. This latter condition is known as a tracheo-oesophageal fistula or TOF for short. The eventual aim of surgery in this situation was to join the two ends of the oesophagus together (or to perform a transplant), so the child could eat normally.

The first documented description of this condition is fascinating. In November 1696, GP Dr Thomas Gibson was called to a house to see a newborn baby who couldn't swallow. Dr Gibson wrote in 1697:

"The child seemed very desirous of food, and took what was offered it in a spoon with greediness: But when it went to swallow it, it was like to be choked, and what should have gone down returned by the mouth and the nose, and it fell into a struggling convulsive sort of fit upon it."

He later reported that the child died and the post-mortem confirmed that the child had a TOF.[37/38]

The first reported case of surgery for this condition was carried out by F.J. Steward at GOS in 1902. The baby survived for 14 days. It wasn't until 1947 that the first two successful repairs of OA were performed by R.H. Franklin at the Hammersmith Hospital. Then in 1948, Denis Browne and Robin Pilcher operated on six babies with the same condition at GOS, three of them surviving.[39]

Although very few of these babies survived in the early years of surgery, by the 1960s 95 per cent were surviving in leading children's hospitals. "This was thanks to astute nurses and midwives recognising the condition earlier and also because their care had improved dramatically," wrote Eoin Aberdeen in 1964.[40/41]

Most babies had died in their first week or two of life from pneumonia caused by secretions (spit) or milk from feeds entering their lungs. By keeping the child's airway clear with intermittent suction, barrier nursing them in incubators and, if their condition allowed, operating early to connect the two ends of the oesophagus, the life expectancy of many of these children was greatly improved.

The child in the buggy that I took an interest in, whom I shall call Rachael, wasn't a straightforward case. She was unable to have early surgery because she had long gap OA, which a very small percentage of these babies have. Long gap OA is difficult to close successfully without the surgeon performing a transplant.

Mr David Waterston, Rachael's surgeon, wrote about her early reconstruction surgery, which involved transplanting a piece of a child's bowel to replace the oesophagus.[41/42] When I met Rachael, she was six months old and waiting for such a transplant operation, too risky to perform in the first weeks of life. This would be her final surgical operation; she'd already undergone a number of operations to keep her alive.

I was so interested in Rachael's condition that I researched what Mr Waterston would have done for her. Her first operation was to close her fistula and prevent the choking fit that Dr Gibson witnessed in 1696 and could have led to Rachael's death. Her second operation was to create an opening out on to Rachael's neck from her oesophagus. From this opening, Rachael's spit and her food and drink would spill out and be caught in a cloth.

I was fascinated at how Rachael was being managed as I had never nursed a child with this rare condition. Rachael was fed normally but the feeding process was called "sham feeding" or pretend feeding. This pretend feeding was very important for Rachael as it was to help her to learn how to feed normally. Without it, she wouldn't have developed the skills to bottle-feed, be weaned, experience tasting, move food around her mouth, chew or swallow and above all, enjoy food.

This wasn't easy work, as sham or pretend feeding is a slow process if it's to be a success. With her "sham feed", Rachael had to have food directly into her stomach so that she also experienced the feeling of having a full stomach while she was tasting and swallowing the food. To achieve this, Mr Waterston had performed a gastrostomy – creating an opening into the stomach through which Rachael could be fed her special nourishing food through a syringe. I witnessed this food being dripped into her stomach in the outpatient department.

It was later, when I'd left the outpatient department, that I learnt that Rachael had had her operation. It was the talk of the hospital. Many of the staff had met her on her outings in her buggy and were impressed with her quick recovery. We learnt that the operation to transplant the piece of bowel had been a success and that Rachael was eating normally. Her split fistula and stomach tube opening had been closed. She was making such good progress that her parents at long last were preparing to take her home. What amazing progress surgery and nursing had made from such dismal beginnings.

After three weeks in general outpatients, I was told that the orthodontic outpatient department had requested my help. They had a bout of staff sickness and wanted an extra pair of hands that I was glad to provide. I'd been a patient of theirs in my first year of training, having that tooth moved into its correct position, and this helped me to know and understand what might be required of me.

While in this unit, I did general chairside assisting, which was rather like being a dental nurse in an ordinary dentist's surgery, finding and passing instruments and assisting in any way I was asked, particularly with babies who had been born with a cleft lip and palate.

Since the early 1950s, it had been routine for babies with clefts of the lip and palate to wear a plate in their mouth, starting soon after birth. I was to assist with the fitting of "Burston McNeil" appliances. These were a series of acrylic plates fitted inside the mouth designed to gradually manipulate the segments of the baby's gum into a more uniform position.[43] The plates were meant to help with feeding by forming a false palate, preventing milk from entering the child's nose passages. This procedure, when accompanied with sticking plaster across the baby's front lip, was meant to make the surgery easier to perform as there was less tension on the lip and would result in a better-looking repair.[44]

The fitting of these plates wasn't a pleasant experience for the mother or baby. To make a mould of the baby's palate, a metal plate containing a plasticine was inserted into the baby's mouth. To do this, I would position the baby on the mother's lap and hold the baby's head in position to ensure they were still enough for the mould to be taken. This made the child gag and very occasionally vomit. The whole procedure had to be repeated regularly as the child grew. I could see that the plates could cause sore areas in the baby's mouth, especially as they began to fit less comfortably. I was encouraged to tell the parents that I had had to wear one of these plates myself but wasn't convinced that this gave much reassurance.

During these final few months of my training, I was travelling daily from our newly-weds' flat in Mortlake, southwest London, and taking a bus and then the Tube to GOS in central London. The work and the commute were exhausting. My last four weeks were spent on relief, working wherever I was needed in the hospital. I was mostly specialling children on wards and on a ventilator. I felt very proud that these children were now entrusted into my care as my seniority and my experience was being recognised.

I remember specialling a baby on 6C&D with congenital hydrocephalus (excess fluid in the brain) after his surgery to insert a Spitz-Holter valve. This device had an interesting beginning. John W. Holter was a machinist for a lock company in Philadelphia when in 1955, his son Casey was born and diagnosed at birth with "water on the brain". A surgeon, Dr Spitz, told John Holter about a shunt (on this occasion, a tube to remove excess fluid from the brain) that he'd devised. He explained that he'd been having problems with the valve of this shunt, so it was likely to fail if he used it on Holter's son. Holter headed home, locked himself up in his garage and three weeks later emerged with the first prototype of what would later be called the Spitz-Holter Shunt.[45]

The first of these valves was inserted at the children's hospital in Philadelphia in March 1956. Mr George Macnab, the consultant paediatric neurosurgeon who taught us in the nursing school and was the surgeon on 6C&D, had worked for years trying to find a solution to the problem of hydrocephalus. Before this surgery, there had been no treatment for this condition. The few children who didn't die during the first years of their life had enormous heads, were blind, deaf, mentally impaired and put into institutions.[46]

Mr Macnab visited Dr Spitz in Philadelphia.[47] He was impressed with the valve and the surgical procedure. Bookvar et al. writing about the development of the Spitz-Holter Shunt in the *Journal of Neurosurgery* in 2001 wrote that: "The valve was patented, Macnab took it back to

England and began using it at GOS, where it became known as the Spitz-Holter Valve. This was groundbreaking surgery. The valve was implanted into an estimated 100,000 people during the 1960s."[48]

In the case of the baby that I specialled (I will call him Ian), this one-way valve had been inserted into his brain by Mr Macnab with the tube draining the extra fluid into the peritoneal cavity of his stomach. Immediately after the operation, I took on the responsibility for his care. I remember the valve of the tube, where the fluid gathered, was located just under the surface of the skin behind Ian's ear. The valve had to be pressed manually a prescribed number of times at intervals during the day to stop the pressure of fluid building up in the brain. This was one of my tasks while I was specialling him.

I specialled Ian for two days, during which I had a number of other procedures to fulfil. He was nursed in a semi-sitting position, the angle of which would be governed by his blood pressure readings. I took these readings every half an hour. If the readings dropped, then lowering his head more would improve them and provide a better supply of blood to the vital centre of his brain.

He had an infusion of fluid into his vein for the first 48 hours. I performed the routine of recording the amount of fluid given every 15 minutes, counting the number of drops going through the chamber and altering the flow if it was incorrect. I took and recorded his pulse and respiration rate, again every 15 minutes, checking that there was no rise or fall in the pulse rate and no irregular or rapid respirations. I recorded his temperature hourly to check that it didn't exceed 102 degrees Fahrenheit.[46] There were no machines to record these vital signs at that time, so all these tasks were labour intensive. This and the general observation and care of a child after surgery, including the regular manual pressing of the Spitz-Holter valve, would have been my role in looking after Ian.

After 48 hours, when Ian's observations were stable and he began to take his regular bottle feeds, I stopped the infusion into his vein and his quarter-hourly observations became four-hourly. My role of 'specialling' him was over and the ward staff took on the responsibility for his care. When Ian had recovered enough to be discharged home, the family and eventually Ian himself had to continue to press this valve regularly for his lifetime. This small inconvenience would mean that he could live a normal life.

We finished our training at the end of September 1966 and had our exit interview with Miss Kirby. Once again, I was back in her office, but there was no need to worry this time.

"Have you enjoyed your training, Nurse Martin?" she asked me.

"Yes, very much so," I replied.

"What are your hopes and plans for the future?"

Matron was always keen that her students should stay on as staff nurses at GOS if they could.

"There's a staff nurse's post at Queen Mary's Hospital in Roehampton and as the hospital is within cycling distance of my home. I've applied."

"In which department is this post?"

"The paediatric burns and plastics unit."

"I hope very much that you enjoy working there," she replied. "Before you go," Matron added, "I have a note here about a thermometer incident. I am planning to delete it from your records. I hope you're happy with that?"

"I am, Matron," I replied.

"I wish you every success for your future," she said.

And that was that. For now.

In October, our group of students sat our registered sick children's finals. We were given a written paper, and a practical examination that was organised by outside examiners. I realised then how little revision I'd managed to do for these finals, but hoped I'd somehow pass them. Soon after this, I found that although I'd passed my practical examination, I'd failed my written one. I was very upset by this, but it was only a temporary setback and I was able to retake it three months later. Thankfully, this time I passed.

In November 1967, all the 1962 sets of students had a presentation day when we received our hospital certificates and our hospital badges. It was a very grand occasion, and the certificates were to be presented to us by Princess Alexandra. Only two of our relatives were invited and as both my parents wanted to come, John volunteered to stay behind.

I remember that we weren't allowed to organise our own uniforms. We were dressed for the occasion and our GOS caps had been specially made up for us in a way that we had never remembered seeing them made up before. They were actually clipped on to our heads for us. When I came to be presented to Princess Alexandra, she singled me out and said that she understood that I had married during my training.

"Did you find getting married at that time hard?" she asked me.

I admitted to her that yes, it was indeed hard, but I wouldn't have had it any other way.

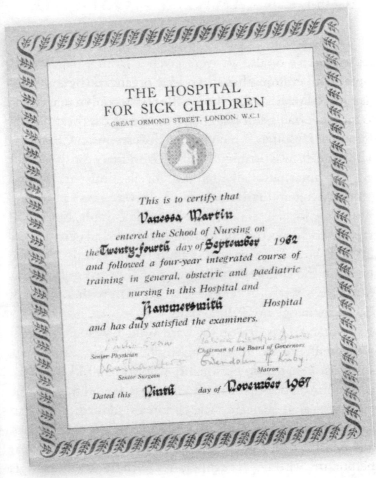

GOS hospital certificate.

QUEEN MARY'S HOSPITAL

In September 1966, I began working as a staff nurse on J Ward at Queen Mary's Hospital, in Roehampton in southwest London. It had been designated as part of the Westminster Group of Hospitals, which included Westminster Children's Hospital. It was originally a huge military hospital but became internationally famous for its limb fitting and amputee rehabilitation centres.[49] It was now a general hospital with adult medical and surgical wards, but it had retained its expertise for treating burns and plastic surgery cases, as well as its specialist limb fitting centre. I was to work on the children's plastic and oral surgery ward. I was fitted for a Westminster Hospital uniform with a different hat to challenge my sewing skills.

I worked day shifts on the ward as there were permanent night staff nurses. Sister Knight who ran the ward was a softly spoken, gentle personality whom we all liked. There were four staff nurses including myself working on the day shift, all registered sick children's trained. I made a particular friend of Gill, who was one of the staff nurses. She had trained at GOS and had started in 1961, the year before me. We'd never met before, which wasn't unusual as there were many staff I never met while working at GOS. The other two staff nurses had qualified at Westminster

Children's Hospital. We all worked well together, but it was always particularly good working with Gill. There were Westminster Hospital students on the ward, training either to become adult-registered nurses or doing their sick children's training, which we had to oversee.

There were also two auxiliary nurses. One of the auxiliary nurses, whom I admired, had previously been nanny to David Attenborough's children. She was so reliable and efficient that it was a pleasure to work with her. I have often thought how interesting it must have been to work for the Attenborough family. Finally, there was a Voluntary Aid Detachment (VAD) nurse, who had been awarded the state enrolled nurse qualification. We didn't have any state enrolled nurses at GOS. Some adult training hospitals took on students to do this two-year training to become practical or bedside nurses. They were invaluable at carrying out normal routine work on patients to enable the staff nurses to manage wards when the sister wasn't around.

VAD nurses had an interesting history. The VAD was a voluntary unit of civilian nurses who provided care for military personnel during both world wars. County branches of the Red Cross had their own groups of Voluntary Aid Detachments, men and women who carried out a range of positions including nursing, transport duties and the organisation of rest stations, working parties, auxiliary hospitals and convalescent homes.

There were about 3,000 temporary auxiliary hospitals across the UK and, like today's Nightingale Hospitals (built to deal with the possible overflow of Covid-19 patients), they were adapted from appropriate buildings, equipped and staffed and ready to be used by wounded servicemen returning from abroad.

Penny Starns, who did a dissertation at Bristol University titled "Military influence on the British civilian nursing profession", says that the military, being part of the established male patriarchal society, denied the volunteer women any form of organised training. Although their model of practice included "early recruitment and the specialist training of cadets in a separate college", they failed to incorporate these features when recruiting female civilians. To alleviate nurse shortages and through the army cadet schemes, "Fifteen-year-old girls were recruited directly from school and expected to perform skilled nursing tasks, often without supervision. In some instances, cadets were responsible for stitching wounds, attending post-mortems and feeding premature babies."[50/51]

J Ward was on the ground floor of the hospital with a garden around it where children could play. The garden had many pedal cars and prams as well as a lovely rocking horse, a favourite of many children.

As the ward served the community, many children were well known to us. One young girl with Apert's syndrome, a combination of symptoms that affected her skull, face, hands and feet, was a frequent visitor. She was having her fused fingers and toes separated and grafted with her own skin so that they functioned better for her. It was a long process, but she knew the staff so well that she seemed to really enjoy her frequent admissions to the ward. She was a joy to look after as she was such a happy child. Her learning disability never slowed her down; she was always playing in the ward garden, especially on the rocking horse, and would

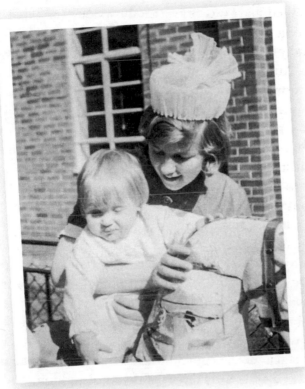

A different child playing on the famous rocking horse, loved by many.

be begging us to go outside to play, rain or shine, even when she had just returned from the operating theatre.

It was good to consolidate my plastic surgery experience from Ward 4C&D at GOS. I enjoyed now being able to take responsibility for the pre- and post-operative nursing care of children with cleft lip and palate, as well as their feeding, which was sometimes challenging.

Although all the staff worked well together, there was one staff member with whom I felt uncomfortable. That was the VAD nurse. I was aware that she was very unhappy about me being in charge of the ward when she was on duty. I was 22 and newly qualified. What did I know about running a ward? After the Second World War, she'd responded to the government's appeal to recruit nursing staff to hospitals. I had no idea of the experience of this VAD nurse as I'd never known her socially, but I knew she'd worked on J Ward for a number of years.

There was one incident which changed our relationship. One evening, we were on a late shift together, working alongside two Westminster students. The shift had been uneventful as most of the children on the ward had been admitted ready for the plastic surgery list the following morning. One of these was a baby listed for the repair of a cleft palate. The VAD nurse had asked to look after this baby, and I understood that she was experienced in looking after babies with a cleft lip and palate.

It was late evening, and the baby was being fed by the VAD nurse in the cubicle next door to the office where I was writing the daily report of the ward children. Suddenly there was frantic banging on the cubicle window. I turned around to see the VAD nurse holding the baby, who was a dark navy colour. I shouted for the students to get the oxygen and suction from the ward cupboard (there was no piped oxygen and suction on the ward) and told the VAD nurse to phone the switchboard for help.

The baby's mouth was full of cereal. I put the baby's face down across my knee and began to remove as much cereal as I could. The students plugged in the machine and I started to suction the baby's nose and mouth. This removed most of the rest of the cereal. I then started mouth-to-mouth resuscitation on the baby. After a while he began coughing and his colour was returning.

I had the oxygen mask on the baby's face when an anaesthetist ran into the cubicle. The switchboard staff had found him on the ward next door. Together we set up an oxygen tent for the baby to sleep in overnight. I knew that one of the part-time night staff nurses liked the occasional extra shift. I arranged for her to special the child for the rest of the night.

The next morning, I came on duty as usual and was met by the consultant plastic surgeon and the same anaesthetist. The surgeon shook my hand and thanked me profusely for what I'd done. He told me that they'd both examined the baby, who appeared fit and well. They would be sending him for a chest X-ray to confirm that his lungs were clear. The surgeon told me that his operation would be postponed for now and he would be discharged home later that day.

After this incident, the VAD nurse treated me quite differently and responded to every request I made. While this made my job a whole lot easier, the incident brought home to me how vulnerable babies with a cleft lip and/or a cleft palate are when being fed. I realised the importance of specialist training on feeding these babies and why trained staff always fed them at GOS.

Christmas was approaching and preparations were under way for the ward party. About 50 children were invited each year to this party. The ward needed to be decorated, the windows painted and Father Christmas organised with presents. There was even a magician and a clown attending. An incredible feast was also being arranged, with contributions from past parents and local firms as well as staff.

Everything was booked and ready by the middle of December, when a child was diagnosed with mumps. The ward had to be closed and disinfected. I still have a copy of the letter that went out to every parent apologising for the cancellation of the party. Apparently, this was the first time that it had ever happened. I'd never had mumps as a child but, luckily, I must have been immune to the infection, as I never came down with it even though it's highly contagious. Another member of staff did contract it and felt dreadful.

The adult plastic surgery ward, the burns unit and the children's plastic surgery ward were next to each other. There was an area where burns patients were admitted as emergencies. We were often asked to help out in this unit, especially when children were admitted.

The most frequent children's admissions were the result of a child grabbing the handle of a pan on a stove. This would cause scalding of an arm and part of the body with boiling water or soup – a very painful injury. I always made sure, when I had children myself and was cooking, that the pan handles on my stove were turned inwards so they were away from inquisitive little hands.

One particular incident I remember was when a family were involved in a house fire. They were on their way to the unit by ambulance. A teenage boy was involved in this fire, and I was asked look after him when he arrived. I'd been in charge of the evening shift on J Ward and was about to go off duty. I stayed on to receive this youngster and perform his emergency treatment.

When he arrived, I was reminded of the five boys I'd looked after on the burns unit at GOS. Luckily this lad had no facial burns. The emergency treatment was similar though. Sedating the child, giving him painkillers and antibiotics, giving him oxygen temporarily by mask and fluids by intravenous infusion were the first priorities. What I remember most was having to gently clean all his deep burns with 1 per cent cetrimide, an antiseptic with cleansing properties. I also had to snip away blisters that were trying to form, before dressing these wounds. Up to now, I'd only ever observed this treatment, but now had to perform it myself. It wasn't a pleasant task, but was essential in those days to ensure the wound was clean and free of infection before the pressure dressings were applied.

At home, John was getting worried about me. We had a 1946 Ford Anglia, which he had bought for £35 before he went to university. His university friends had named her Jehu because "Jehu drove his chariot furiously".[52] Often he couldn't afford to run the car, but with two incomes, we were trying to keep it on the road. He'd phoned the hospital and found out that I was held up looking after an emergency burns case. When I'd finished with this young boy, he was waiting outside for me in the car. I left my bicycle at the hospital that night and John dropped me off for my next shift the following morning.

It was during my holiday that year that I concentrated on my driving skills. I was encouraged to drive to Scotland and back, as Carol (who had moved permanently to Scotland) had invited us to stay with her. A few weeks after I returned from my holiday and with my newly found confidence, I took my driving test in Jehu. Luckily, I passed first time and was able to tease John as he had to take it three times.

It was soon after this that I discovered I was pregnant with my first child. Christmas wasn't far away and thankfully, there was no mumps on J Ward this year. The party was held during the week before Christmas, and Father Christmas, the magician and the clown came to entertain the children. It was well attended by both children and their parents, as well as nursing and medical staff.

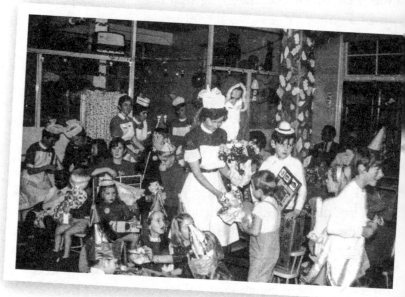

A presentation of thanks to Sister Knight.

The ward was kept open over Christmas and the New Year for emergency admissions with just a skeleton staff. I worked on Christmas Day (as did John) to allow other staff to be with their families and had Boxing Day at home. It was a quiet Christmas compared to the ones I'd experienced at GOS, but still enjoyable.

I'd already handed in my notice by now. At that time, if you became pregnant, it was expected that you left your place of work to concentrate on bringing up your child. There was no maternity leave or maternity pay. I left the ward in January after a small leaving party. The VAD nurse slipped me a personal present, a Wedgwood Beatrix Potter Peter Rabbit plate and cup set for my new baby. It was a beautiful and flattering reminder that people can surprise you.

Jonathan was born at Queen Mary's Hospital in March 1968. I had wonderful care. It wasn't routine then to have your husband with you at the birth, but John was allowed to support me because they knew me as a member of staff. It made so much difference to us that our son's birth had been a shared experience.

Jonathan fed well, gained weight and his early development was normal. What he didn't do was sleep very much. At night, four hours was the most you could hope for. He was a happy child when well fed, but he played and giggled all night, keeping John and I awake. We found we couldn't sleep with him. We only had one bedroom in our ground-floor flat, so the only option was for us was to move into our front room. We had a couch that pulled out into a double bed where we slept. In the daytime, we stored our double sleeping bag and pillows behind it. The problem with this front room was not only was it our living room, but John used it as a study, writing sermons and interviewing wedding couples there. To add to the chaos, once a week we ran one of the church youth clubs in this room, entertaining up to 12 teenagers. It was hard work keeping it tidy.

Jonathan was baptised when he was three months old. We invited John's father to baptise him. Gill and her husband, my school friend Carol and John's brother were godparents. We had a celebration tea in the church hall as there was no way we could entertain in our tiny flat.

LIFE IN BERMONDSEY

In 1969, John was invited to become the missioner at the Charterhouse School Mission. He accepted the role and we moved to Bermondsey, just south of London Bridge and Guy's Hospital. He'd been attracted to the job because he felt that the role of British missionaries abroad was becoming less influential as they were foreigners and the indigenous Christians were much more effective. The inner cities of Britain were now the mission fields and where the church was struggling. In fact, we soon discovered that in these areas, the whole community was struggling.

We moved into a building owned and financed by the Charterhouse School Mission. They employed a cook and a cleaner for the building, which contained two flats, one for the missioner and the other for a youth club leader. There were also rooms that were rented out to students. We were expected, if requested, to entertain any "old boy" or visitor from Charterhouse School, which was why the cook was employed. She provided a delicious midday meal on weekdays in the dining room at a long refectory table. Both the cook and the cleaner refused to eat with us, so John would be served his meal at one end of the table and I, with Jonathan in his highchair, at the other end.

It wasn't long before John decided that if they wouldn't

join us to eat, we would join them in the kitchen. They were horrified when we walked into their kitchen with our plates and promptly moved into the dining room to eat with us. That continued unless we had an important visitor – a rare occurrence – when they'd insist on waiting on them.

Our building was in Tabard Street, not far from Borough Underground station. Diagonally opposite us was a large block of flats, Chaucer House, Southwark's home for the homeless. It had been provided in response to the 1966 BBC play *Cathy Come Home*. The drama has been named as "UK's most influential programme of all time" and had highlighted the plight of homeless families.[53] Chaucer House was innovative at the time because fathers could stay with their wives and children. Lambeth Council had a similar homeless unit in the area. Chaucer contained 100 families and 400 children. When I tried to have a daily paper delivered to us, I was refused because of where we lived.

The area became particularly noisy and active at night. One morning, someone was brought to our door who had been stabbed, and John had to call an ambulance. He was very protective of Jonathan and me and wouldn't allow me to take our car to the Charterhouse rented garage nearby after dark. I had to leave it on the pavement outside our building for him to park. The car was now a three-wheel Reliant, an older model than the one seen in *Only Fools and Horses*.

My health visitor never visited me at home as she knew I was a paediatric nurse, but we used to see each other in the street. She always said to me that if I had any problems, I would be welcome to contact her. I was actually beginning to have some concerns.

At the age of two years Jonathan had a large vocabulary, but he wasn't yet forming them into sentences. At night he still only slept for four and a half hours and was constantly on the go. In every other way his development was normal, to the extent that one night at Easter, he'd gone into the room where we had a tall, decorative sideboard. He moved a chair and climbed onto the sideboard, then onto a small shelf in order to reach the family's Easter eggs that I'd hidden six feet from the ground. He ate the lot. He was 13 months old. He showed us how he managed to climb up!

After I spoke to my health visitor, she referred him to a paediatrician at nearby Guy's Hospital, Professor Robinson. He took great trouble with Jonathan, first observing him in their play area and then doing various tests on him. He even took blood and a skin sample for genetic testing. All Jonathan's results were within normal parameters. Professor Robinson concluded that Jonathan was just hyperactive, was too busy to sleep and wasn't concentrating for long enough to think about forming his words into sentences.

It was soon after that, in September 1970, that James was born at Guy's Hospital. This was nothing like the wonderful experience I'd had at Queen Mary's Hospital. It was a huge struggle to have John present and the midwife was very rough with me. I was told by the obstetrician who stitched me up that I had a second-degree tear. James was a bonny baby though; he was contented and slept throughout the night. After more than two years of sleepless nights with Jonathan, this was such a relief for both John and me.

After this, I was at home looking after the two children. I began to feel that I could contribute some of my time to the community. John suggested that I might like to run a young mothers' group once a week in the small hall inside our building. A play group was already running in the hall three days a week. Church members were enthusiastic and keen to help me, so I began to advertise in local shops. Gradually, we began to get more mothers and their children, including some from Chaucer House.

It was fascinating getting to know these mothers and learning about the circumstances that led to them becoming homeless. I met and became friendly with Valerie, who was married to a Cypriot and mother to two delightful boys. She invited me back to her flat in Chaucer House for coffee. I was appalled at the conditions in which the families there were expected to live. There was one outside toilet for four flats, and no bathroom. The kitchen had the only supply of water, with a large stone sink where the family washed the dishes and themselves.

Valerie showed me the state of the oven that was supplied. She'd tried to clean it but it was covered with years of burnt food and inches of grease. It made me feel quite sick to look at it, let alone the thought of cooking food in it. How long would I survive living in these conditions? John and I discussed it. Probably no more than three months, we thought. But families were often in those flats for two years before being rehoused.

I learned a bit about why Valerie and her family were in Chaucer House. Her husband had a full-time job which made me more curious. It turned out they'd been renting a home in the area, but it was repossessed. They tried very hard to rent another one but were constantly refused by landlords because her husband was a Turkish Cypriot.

"We landed up as a family on the streets," Valerie told me. "We didn't know what to do. It was awful. We went to the council and they sent us here."

"What about your own family?"

"There's just my dad."

"Do you see much of him? Couldn't he help?"

"We see him regularly, but he doesn't know we're here. I daren't tell him. I don't want to. We need to be self-sufficient." She lowered her voice. "He's a local councillor."

We continued to meet regularly outside the young mothers' group and I found out more about Valerie. Every morning when it was time for the children to go to the nearby primary school, Valerie would knock on the doors along her balcony. She'd collect and take all her neighbours' children along with her own.

"The problem I had at the beginning was that some of the children are short of clothes. I went to East Lane market and bought some very cheap items, including gloves and hats. I'm particularly worried about the girls having no pants, so I bought a pack and I make sure they're wearing a pair before I take them to school."

What I found about having coffee in Valerie's flat was that even though her home was spotless, the children and I always came home smelling really unpleasant. It's hard to explain, but the whole building was permeated with a sort of body odour. It was only after I had bathed us all and washed our clothes that I could get rid of the smell. I remember other people saying to me that it doesn't cost much for people like that to buy a bar of soap. But in my experience of Chaucer House, it wasn't just about keeping your family clean, the smell was part of the fabric of the building itself. There was nothing anyone could do about it.

After two years of living in Chaucer House, I realised how depressed Valerie was becoming. When one day she wouldn't answer the door to me, John and I were really concerned. Chaucer House had an office on the ground floor with 10 social-work students and two senior social workers. John went to the office and spoke to one of the senior social workers, who agreed that Valerie and her family had been coping well until then. The social worker encouraged John to raise their case with the housing department. Not long after that Valerie came to see me. She was delighted that her family had been offered a terraced council house in the borough. I was thrilled for them.

There was another woman, Dora, who came to the young mothers' group. She always stood apart from the other mothers, and never mixed with anyone. Her three-year-old daughter would stand quietly beside her. I tried to talk to Dora, but it was hard to get a conversation going, so I was surprised when one evening she knocked on my door.

"Dora? Hello."

"Hello, Vanessa."

"Come in," I said.

Her daughter was with her, so I found some things for her to play with and I made some coffee.

As we chatted, Dora began to talk. I learnt that she had been fostered as a baby. Her last foster parents had been a Scottish minister and his wife, with whom she was very happy. I didn't push her for more information that day but made it clear that she could come to see me at any time.

She came on several occasions and became more relaxed in my company. She always came with her daughter at a time when my children were in bed. Often her partner would knock on the door later, looking for her. Because it was late, John was around and would say that Dora wasn't ready to see him yet. He'd sit on the steps in the enclosed porch and chat with him.

One evening Dora came to see me and brought with her a carved wooden fish.

"Will you keep this safe for me?" she said.

It seemed like a strange thing to ask me. Then she told me why.

"He does this to me," she said. Before I could say anything, she pulled aside her blouse and showed me her bruises. "He hits me in places where no one else can see them." She then opened the fish that she wanted me to look after.

"It was a present from my foster parents."

It had a catch on the top and opened up to reveal a sharp metal carving knife and fork.

"Please hang onto this for me," she asked again.

"Of course," I said.

"One day he'll kill me with it."

Soon after, Dora told me in confidence that she and her daughter were to be rehoused. The next day they were to go to a secret location. They would stay there overnight until they could be transported to their new lodgings.

"Would you take us there tomorrow, Vanessa? You're the only person I can trust."

I agreed, and we arranged to meet the next day.

I drove the car to our meeting place. She was waiting with her daughter and a small bag with all their belongings.

To anyone else, it might look like she was just out shopping. They got in the car and she gave me directions.

She guided me to what I discovered was a small psychiatric unit. We went in through the doors and she was obviously expected.

"Which one of you is the patient?"

She was thrilled to think that they might have mistaken me for her. Her room was in the male wing of the unit and I was concerned for her and her child. There were a few disturbed patients who were fascinated with both of them. Dora tried not to show me her fear, saying that she would wedge the door with a chair. I left her there, hoping the staff would look after her and that social services would move her quickly from that place.

A few days later, John was taking his usual shortcut through Chaucer House to the church. A group of social workers were in a huddle in the grounds of the flats, and he asked them what was happening. They told him that Dora's boyfriend was still in her flat and they wanted to clear it for a new family to move into.

"Oh, I know him," John said. "I'll go up and see him. Maybe I can help."

He found the boyfriend sitting in the living room on a pile of cases.

"Hello," John said. "I gather the people downstairs want to get in here. Can I give you a hand with these?" He picked up a couple of cases and Dora's boyfriend picked up the others and they took them down to the boyfriend's car, an old banger. They loaded the car, John said "cheerio" and the boyfriend drove off.

A couple of days later John received a letter from the

head of the social work department thanking him for his help. The next time he saw the senior social worker, he told him about the letter and asked him what that was all about.

"Don't you know?" asked the social worker. "Dora's boyfriend was a member of the Richardsons' gang."

"The Richardsons?"

"Yes. They've been known to nail people to the floor through their knees."

At that time the Richardsons and the Krays were believed to control most of the crime in the East End of London. Fortunately, John hadn't stopped to think. He just knew the boyfriend and thought he could help. The boyfriend responded to his expectations.

I never heard from Dora again, but the social workers told us that she'd been rehoused some distance away and was very happy there. I would have liked to have returned the fish to her (I still have it), but she was in a secret location so that was not possible.

WORKING IN THE COMMUNITY

Valerie and Dora hadn't grown up in the East End of London so didn't speak like typical East Enders. On one occasion a radio service was organised in our church and I was asked to read a lesson. Without any intention of disrespecting our monarch, my new Bermondsey friends told me that I read "like the bleedin' queen"! Later they went to great trouble trying to teach me how to speak to local tradesmen in the East Lane Market, so that I could get the best price for the goods they were selling.

The mission ran a Boys' Club and employed a leader to run it. The club included a gym and was open most of the week for boys to attend. We knew that the Boys' Club leader had occasionally taken boys in the summer for holidays to Charterhouse School in Godalming, Surrey, to camp in their scout hall. One year we were invited to take a mixed group of local youngsters there, including some from Chaucer House, for a two-week holiday.

The Boys' Club leader, Bill, John and I were to be in charge of this group. The social workers allocated the children to come on this holiday, organising the appropriate forms and permissions. The form included the question "Does your child ever wet the bed at night?". This had to be answered before social services would let the children go on holiday. We were asked to take a particularly "at risk" twelve-year-old girl from Chaucer House. They were keen for us to report back on how she was during this holiday.

There were two large central rooms in the scout hut, one used as a dormitory for the boys and the other for the girls. John and I had a cornered-off area in the girls' dormitory with mattresses for us and our boys.

For that whole two weeks I wasn't allowed to look after my children. "We're going to give you a break," the girls insisted. They did everything for our boys, from getting them up and dressed in the mornings, feeding them and changing James's nappy, to entertaining them and putting them to bed at night. They were incredibly efficient at these roles and obviously had a lot of practice looking after younger siblings at home as they came from large families. I'd organised the food, but everyone else helped with the preparation of picnics and cooking on the BBQ.

The "at risk" girl was one of the most helpful. We found that two of the younger boys did, in fact, wet the bed. We realised that the stress of living in Chaucer House was delaying the development of some of these children. When she realised what had happened, this girl was quick to take out their camp beds and wash them down. She would leave them to dry in the sun during the day.

During the second week, we visited a convenience store in Godalming. Here they sold pop socks, which were all the rage then. We found out later that three of the girls had stolen some of these pop socks. One of the lads must have told Bill, because after our evening meal he confronted the girls. In fact, he really laid into them in front of us all. John and I weren't happy with how he handled the situation, but we couldn't intervene at that moment.

At about two o'clock in the morning, I heard a noise in the girls' dormitory. In the darkness, I could make out that John and the boys were still asleep, so I got up to see what was going on. As I crossed the room, I saw the three girls trying to climb out of the window.

"Where are you going?" I spoke quietly because I didn't wish to wake up anyone else.

"We're off!" one of them said.

"Where to?" I replied.

They told me they were going home.

These girls weren't retiring; they were tough and streetwise. I knew that they were angry with Bill.

"Let's find a place where we can talk about this," I said.

We went into the kitchen and they sat down. They looked sullen.

"How were you going to get home?" I asked.

"We'd have thumbed," they said.

"That would have been terribly dangerous."

Then I asked them if they were concerned because Bill had ticked them off in front of their mates.

"Yeah," one said.

No amount of reassurance from me was going to make them change their minds and stay and confront them. Eventually I said to them, "What if you took the pop socks back to the shop? What would your mates think of that?"

One of them said, "They'd never believe we'd done that."

"Then let's do it," I replied.

We arranged that I would set an alarm for seven o'clock so that we could leave before everyone else was up and about. We would walk down to the shop together and return the socks. In the morning, the girls were up and dressed before me and we slipped out of the scout hall and walked into Godalming.

The girls waited outside while I went into the shop to talk to the lady who owned it. I explained about the group of children and that the girls needed to return the socks they had stolen. At first she didn't understand what we were trying to do or why. She was so concerned about these girls that she kept saying, "It's OK, let them keep the socks," but she eventually got the message that they needed to do this to save face with their friends.

I brought the girls into the shop and they apologised as we had agreed they should. The lady was lovely to them and not only thanked them for returning the socks but gave them each a packet of biscuits to take home. The others back at the camp were amazed about what they did, and even Bill congratulated them. They felt that they had re-established their reputations. I wished we could have bought pop socks for all the girls. I knew it was hard for them to have to accept that other parents were able to buy things for their children that their parents couldn't afford.

After we returned home to London, the girls came to my door with a bunch of flowers and called out, "Thanks, love!" and ran away. Only slowly did I realise the source of the gift. They'd been growing in a local council flower bed.

Some of the boys came to say thank you too. "Want some paint, Vic?" one of them asked.

"Paint?" John was surprised. "Where would it come from?"

"Found this flat where the council keeps some stuff. It's easy to get in."

"What do your parents think about that?" He asked.

"They've got some too."

John thanked the boys for their generosity but said we didn't need paint just then. We did feel honoured that we were regarded as mates.

Because we lived near the Old Kent Road, close to Borough Market and London Bridge, we were a convenient stopping place for rough sleepers on the hunt for something to eat. Our cook would make up sandwiches for them when she was on duty. Otherwise, when they came to the door, we would give them sandwiches and tea or coffee, but never money. There was also always a good supply of clothes provided by Charterhouse old boys. We had a large chest in the hallway containing underwear, socks, shirts, trousers and pullovers, some of them even new.

I remember one very cold winter's day, John giving his own duffle coat to a man living on the street. I remonstrated with him as not only did he like that coat, but we were quite short of money at the time as I wasn't working. John said that he couldn't bear to turn the man out onto the streets without a coat. When I said that he might just sell it, John said that it was a risk we had to take.

We got to know several men who slept on the streets and visited us regularly. They were known as "tramps" in the 1970s, not to be confused with the homeless, who were rehoused families. John would sit and talk to them and try to find out why they were on the streets. It was often because of a marriage break-up or losing a job. Sometimes they were chaps coming out of the forces, not able to cope without the structure of army discipline, or perhaps they'd been institutionalised in orphanages or prisons.

They got to know that I was a nurse and would constantly complain to me about their sore feet. When I saw their feet, I realised how much walking they must do, often in poorly fitting shoes. They not only had blisters but sometimes quite nasty infected sores. I'd soak their feet in a bowl of warm soapy water, which they liked. Once they were clean and softened, I'd get them to cut their own toenails and then dressed any wounds they had. Finally, I'd make sure they had new, clean socks. It was a small thing, but they always appreciated it.

One day, a young local boy aged 17, called Ted, came to our door. He'd not long left school and had been thrown out of his home by his stepfather. John brought him inside our building to talk to him.

"Where are you living, Ted?"

He confirmed what John thought, that he didn't have a home.

But then Ted surprised him. He said that he wanted to become a Christian and to change his life around.

"If you really want to do that, Ted, I'll help you find a job and a place to live," John said. "But the deal is that you let me run your life for you." Ted was uncertain about this, so John explained: "Well, I'll tell you when to get up in the morning and when to go to bed at night, where to live and I'll find you a job." Ted agreed. "Leave it with me, Ted, and I'll get back to you once I've had a talk with my wife."

So, after a discussion with me and the students living with us, we agreed that we could allow Ted to stay temporarily in one of our student rooms. John also met with our local police to discuss the risk of allowing Ted to live in our building. They said that as long as it wasn't a formal arrangement with him paying rent and having a rent book, we could turn him out at any time if there was trouble.

So, over the next weeks, John went with Ted and found a job for him and, with some charity money, paid a deposit and the first week's rent for a bedsit with a bathroom and cooking facilities for Ted to move into. The time came for Ted to leave us and to start his job. His room was ready.

That night Ted went out and got very drunk. He came back in the early hours of the morning and was obviously having a meltdown about leaving us. He was running up and down the stairs shouting and constantly ringing our doorbell, which was a very loud one. I was worried about our boys. He was also disturbing the students. John went out to talk to him. He warned Ted a number of times that if he continued to cause a rumpus, he would call the police. Ted carried on and John was as good as his word.

Two policemen arrived in a Black Mariah with a pair of Alsatian dogs. When they came into the house, Ted was pleading with John not to let them take him away, his arms clamped around John's legs, sobbing. It was heartbreaking, but there was no turning back. He was escorted out and put in the Black Mariah. Before they left, the officers went upstairs and searched Ted's room. There was more commotion and shouting and we were astonished when we saw the police escorting another man down the stairs.

"We found this one asleep underneath Ted's bed," one of the policemen said.

"Ted's brother," the other one added.

They put him in the van too and, after they left, John and I went back to bed and lay awake for some time, reflecting on what had just happened.

The next day John went to the police station and collected Ted to take him to his new bedsit. Ted was very subdued but he went with him. The sad thing was that not only did Ted give up his job after a week, but he also gave up his bedsit. Ted's problem was that he couldn't cope with relating to people and he really needed a substitute parent or parents to replace what had been missing in his childhood.

Ted came back on a number of occasions asking for a sandwich and a cup of tea. After one visit, he returned to our building asking for John. He'd stolen a tin by our house phone known as the "honesty box", used by the students to put money into for calls. The box was still sealed, the money still in it. Ted told John that he couldn't take money from us, which impressed us. At that time John's stipend was £20 a week. Ted told him he made about £16 a week conning other clergymen out of money.

Ted continued regular visits to our home for a sandwich and a cup of tea and he was always welcomed. Two years later, we moved to another Bermondsey parish, St Anne's, which was beyond Tower Bridge. We lived in a vicarage built into a square of flats that surrounded the church. Ted continued to call by for his sandwich and cuppa. He would tell us that his time with us was the happiest in his life and would often ask if we would put him up again. Even if we wanted to, we had no room for Ted, because we were in a small modern vicarage. We had neither the space nor the time to give him the attention he needed. We couldn't be substitute parents and sadly we knew of no one else who could offer him that relationship.

Ted's health deteriorated fast. He was losing his teeth and those that remained were black. When he began to drink methylated spirits, we knew this was the beginning of the end. I thought of the young man who'd spent his last days on the ward at the Hammersmith. The one whose companions had done their very best to make his last days count. I knew there was nothing we could do.

Eventually Ted stopped visiting and we feared he had died. We had no way of knowing for certain, though I've thought about him many times over the years.

St Anne's parish was only a couple of miles down the road from Charterhouse. It was two communities away, with rows of small, terraced houses. The impressive Victorian church had a newly built square of flats around it with a vicarage set into one corner. The vicarage was a three-storey building with a large study, kitchenette, toilet and garage on the ground floor.

We had six neighbours, three either side, and we lived almost on top of each other. The walls were so thin that we could hear their loos flushing, and no doubt they could hear ours.

After we moved in, we were a magnet to local youngsters who kept knocking on our door and running away. One day I hid behind the door and when a group of them knocked, I chased them into the refuse area, where they were hiding behind the rubbish bins.

"Would you like to come in for coffee?" I asked.

One by one they came out from behind the bins and looked at me in surprise.

"Yeah, Miss," they said and followed me back inside the vicarage.

That was the beginning of the formation of our church youth club.

A group of between eight and 12 youngsters came to our house every Tuesday evening and we did different activities with them. John was good at telling them ghost stories. They loved these so much that John invited the diocesan exorcist to come and talk to them about what to do if they met an actual ghost.

We had regular "Taste and Die" evenings when they each cooked something and we risked our lives eating it! When we had tasted the dishes, we'd vote for the best one. One youngster was notorious for bringing a sliced boiled egg and offering us each a slice to taste.

Then there were occasional outings, as Jonathan's nursery schoolteacher babysat for me once a week to give me a break. We took them to see *Jesus Christ Superstar* at the cinema and to two musicals, *The Witness* in St Martin-in-the-Fields and *Godspell* in Westminster Cathedral. They were blown away by these last two experiences and the magnificence of these two famous churches.

They formed a choir in the church and liked dressing up in robes. I taught two or three of them the basics of playing the guitar. One talented girl had taught herself the piano and we had Nigerian twins in the group who were great on percussion. We occasionally played for a service when we didn't have an organist. We had a link with the Royal School of Church Music (RSCM), which invited us one Saturday to Addington Palace (used as their headquarters), to take part in a demonstration of different types of church music. We played "The Gospel Train" and "Silver Trumpet", for which we were honoured with a rousing round of applause.

Afterwards, the RSCM director, Martin, took everyone into one of their impressive rooms, where an equally impressive buffet was laid out. Our youngsters helped themselves to the buffet and then proceeded to take doggy bags out of their pockets and began to fill them with food as Martin and John were watching.

"I'm so sorry," John said, mortified at their behaviour.

"Please don't worry, John." Martin tried to reassure him. "Listen to me, everyone. I think you'll all agree this is a delicious spread, but we need to make sure there's enough to go around." He then told the youngsters exactly what they could and couldn't take home. He was very understanding.

One evening at youth club I asked the youngsters if they'd like me to make them a posh meal. Many of the council houses where they lived were two-up-two-down: a living room and kitchen downstairs, two bedrooms upstairs and an outside loo. Consequently, families ate their meals while watching the television in the living room, never around a table.

They were keen on my idea and were told to come dressed up, with the boys wearing ties (which came in their pockets). I prepared a four-course meal with a starter, main meal, sweet, and cheese and biscuits. John instructed the boys on how to pull back the chairs for the girls to be seated and showed them how to use their napkins. He poured non-alcoholic drinks into wine glasses. As I served each course, I taught them which set of cutlery to use, just as my grandmother had once shown me. Buttering their bread on my tablecloth was not allowed; it was to be done on their side plates or not at all.

After this evening, our parish was invited to go to Tenterden in the heart of the Weald of Kent, where St Anne's had a link church. Each year, they would invite our congregation to their parish for a day in the country. We would eat a picnic they provided at lunch time and the parishioners took us into their homes for an evening meal. Some youngsters came and were invited in pairs into homes to have an evening meal. It was quite an experience for them. On the coach home, they went up to John and told him that it was good we had taught them their manners. We were glad that they had felt able to cope.

Jonathan, our eldest, had always been active. At four and a half, he still only ever slept for four and a half hours a night. We put a gate in the doorway of his bedroom, which mostly confined him to his room at night, but he crashed about every evening, demolishing his bed and playing until he was exhausted. He would fall asleep wherever he was. Our church youngsters were amazing with him. They got used to him crashing about upstairs and often tried to sneak a peek at him when they used the toilet next door to his room. One Tuesday evening, one of the girls found him asleep and they all trouped upstairs one by one to see this unusual spectacle.

PHILIPPA JOINS THE FAMILY

Life was changing again. I was due to have my third child in January 1973. One night, I knew that I was starting to go into labour, but I also knew that John had all the clergy from the area gathering at St Anne's Church for a service. Though sheer willpower, I managed to hold on until the morning, when things only got more chaotic.

John was making his preparations while I was trying to get the boys up and dressed. I had decided to take them both in the car down to Jonathan's nursery rather than walking. I managed to get them both into the car and the car out of the garage between contractions. I got Jonathan very late to the nursery and told Phyllis, who was Jonathan's teacher, that I was in labour.

She immediately took both boys from me and said, "We'll look after James as well as Jonathan for as long as you need us to. Don't worry, just get yourself to the hospital."

By the time I'd found a parking space outside Guy's Hospital and managed to walk into the maternity unit, it was past lunch time. I told the midwives at the desk that this was my third child and I was approaching my second stage of labour, but they were sceptical.

One of them said, "I'll take you and examine you. That will put your mind at rest."

I'd hardly been on the couch when the midwife rushed out, and she and her colleague ran back with a trolley. With great speed they transferred me to the labour suite. I'd been worried about returning to Guy's Hospital for the birth because of my experience with James.

This time the midwife approached me and surprised me by saying, "I can assure you, Mrs Martin, that the midwife you had before will not be looking after you. She's not on duty. I promise you that we will take good care of you."

They kept their promise and were wonderful to me. I'd told them that John didn't even know that I was in hospital, and they assured me that they had contacted him and he was on his way. As men were beginning to be with their wives during birth, John was welcomed. He was by my side just in time to see Philippa arrive into the world at 3.30 in the afternoon. I needed no stitches this time.

I'd really wanted a girl, so I was thrilled when Philippa was born. She was beautiful and the boys adored her. They took turns in holding her and Jonathan loved stroking her hair. She also slept really well at night, which was wonderful.

Considering Bermondsey was such a deprived area of London, it surprisingly had the most amazing nursery, to which I'd taken both of my boys. It was a service provided by Southwark and was extremely efficiently run by the principal, Miss Furneaux. The children had daily formal lessons as well as lots of outdoor play. They all loved being there. Jonathan needed a firm hand in nursery as he could be quite disruptive but Phyllis, his teacher, was wonderful with him and knew exactly how to distract him if he had a tantrum.

Professor Robinson, the paediatrician at Guy's Hospital, had been seeing Jonathan occasionally to keep an eye on his progress. He told John and I that he would try Jonathan on a small dose of Ritalin, a central nervous system stimulant that was being trialled. He said he could only give us this one trial course as it hadn't yet been licensed. Jonathan was much more alert and co-operative while taking this medicine. This excited us, but it was only temporary. He was only on the drug for two weeks and wasn't allowed to have a repeat prescription.

Miss Furneaux liaised with the local church primary school when Jonathan was five. It was agreed that he should stay at Kintore Way Nursery for an extra year so that we could organise an extra support teacher, funded by a charity, to work with him in the classroom. As this was the year that Philippa was born and James was approaching three, he was offered a place at the nursery and I was able to take both boys to Kintore Way, walking with Philippa in the pram. Phyllis found it useful to have James around as he kept an eye out for Jonathan and told her if he was misbehaving.

James was the organiser and negotiator and was always alert to everything that went on around him. When James was four, John had a couple coming for an interview with him one afternoon before their wedding. John was in the downstairs toilet and the couple came to the door early for their appointment. James was playing on the staircase to our flat above.

John said to him, "James, would you open the front door and show these two into my study? Tell them I will be with them shortly."

James did as he was told. He politely showed the couple

into the study and told them that his daddy would be with them soon, but then added, "He's on the toilet, wiping his bottom."

John heard it all. He then had to go and greet the couple and chat to them about their wedding as if nothing untoward had been said.

Later during our time at St Anne's, a gentleman came to our front door and told John that he had just moved into a flat next door to us.

"Could I borrow a chair?" he asked John.

"Of course," John replied. "I'll carry it up for you."

When he walked through the door of the flat, John was horrified to find that, except for a pile of newspapers on the floor where the gentleman slept, the place was completely bare.

"I've been homeless," the gentleman told John. "Recently, I've been staying in a Salvation Army hostel. A few years ago, I was advised to go on the waiting list for a council property. Now finally I've got a flat of my own."

"Do social services know you've got no furniture?" John asked.

"No," the man said.

"Right, well, it's Friday night. I can't contact them now until Monday. Leave it with me."

In the notices at the church service on Sunday morning, John mentioned to our small congregation that this gentleman had moved in next door to us and asked if they had anything in the way of spare furniture to help him until he could contact social services. The response was so incredible that we were left speechless.

By Sunday evening the flat was not only fully furnished and a bed made up for him, but people had donated their spare curtains and hung them in the windows, someone had found a cooker and another a fridge in which they had put milk, bread, margarine and some basic food. Someone even provided him with an evening meal. And it didn't stop there. On evenings that followed, I saw various people dropping in a casserole or a cake for him. The people among whom we lived in Bermondsey had very little themselves but were extremely generous with what they had.

As for myself, I didn't see much of this gentleman out and about as he wasn't a sociable person, but John saw him regularly. Every evening when he came in late, John told me that he would spot the gentleman standing at the bottom of his staircase, watching our house. As soon as John arrived home, he'd disappear back to his flat.

"Why does he do that?" I asked John.

"I know he's worried about you being at home alone with three children," he told me. "He's keeping an eye on you all until I get home."

Recently, we met together with some of the family. James's wife was there and she said she knew this story because James had told her that he'd been there when the gentleman called. James said he remembered his dad finding a chair and that he'd gone up to the flat with John. (We were thunderstruck. John had no recollection that four-year-old James was with him.) James, now 47 years later, tells us that seeing this empty flat at such an early age and someone living in such poverty had a profound effect on him.

"I was shocked that someone would live in a home with nothing in it and that he would have to sleep on newspaper.

I remember him telling Dad that he wanted the chair so that he could sit and look out of the window. I felt it was so sad that that was all he had to do – sit and look out of a window on a borrowed chair."

A little later James told me that he often thinks of this man, especially when someone remarks that there's no poverty in Britain.

His comment to them is: "Next door to you could live someone who could die in poverty and you wouldn't know about it. Government policies today should all revolve around the people most in need."

Jonathan went to St James' Church of England Primary School when he was six. The school was amazing with him, and the children, who knew he had special needs, took a lot of trouble including him in their games. His speech was improving, and we were pleased that he was beginning to conform to the school routine.

Jonathan's support teacher was amazing too. She was able to help Jonathan to concentrate and commit to different tasks. He was definitely learning and progressing in the school. His reading was improving and his writing becoming more legible. It was his maths that we noticed the most. He was very interested in numbers and keen to do addition and subtraction in his head when asked. We were so pleased with how the school was supporting and developing our son.

He'd been there a year when the headmistress called us to her office and said that she was disappointed to find that the Inner London Education Authority were worried about creating a precedent by keeping Jonathan in a standard primary school. It wasn't their policy and they feared that other parents would demand similar support. They'd told her that she couldn't keep him at the school. We were very upset, and so was she. We were to have a visit from the educational psychologist, Dr Rabinovitz, who would decide with us where Jonathan should go.

Dr Rabinovitz met us at home and asked us many questions, mostly about us, our family life and then later, Jonathan. During this inquisition I couldn't help but reflect on Mildred Creake's comments to us at Great Ormond Street – how children's psychological problems were generally thought to be caused by their parents' inadequacies.

"Are you assessing Jonathan, or us as parents?" I asked eventually.

I could see he was embarrassed at this. He didn't deny that he'd been assessing us.

Eventually he said, "I can offer Jonathan a school for the educationally subnormal, a school for delicate children, or an autistic school."

Those were our choices and it was clear which one was the most appropriate. Jonathan didn't lack intelligence, nor was he delicate by any stretch of the imagination, so we opted for the autistic school. He hadn't been diagnosed with autism, but this school offered the highest academic teaching standards. Nowadays we would be offered support in a primary school, though getting that support might be an issue.

So, in 1975, when Jonathan was seven, he was sent to the Sybil Elgar School in Ealing, London. He was collected every morning and returned to us in the evening. We had regular feedback on his performance and found that he kept trying to fool them into thinking he could do less than he was capable of doing. His maths was always brilliant, and he could read well for his age. When they realised this, they began to stretch him more.

What was worrying us, though, was that he was losing his speech. When he was at St James' School, he was always being stimulated to speak by his peers. This wasn't happening at Sybil Elgar school. Whenever we visited him, he would be sitting with the other children in silence. Another thing we noticed was that he was displaying some very odd behaviour that we'd never seen him do before. He was punching the air, shaking his head and twitching. We put it down to the fact that he must be copying the behaviour of some of the other children in the school. We were glad to have him home in the evenings and at weekends as he was particularly fond of his brother and sister. We felt they had influence over him and could encourage him to be more sociable.

In 1976, when Philippa was three years old, she was also offered a full-time place at Kintore Way. One of the elderly ladies, Maud, who lived across the square from us volunteered to look after her in the event that we needed additional childcare. Because Philippa really liked her, I decided to explore the possibility of returning to my nursing career.

I'd been out of nursing for eight years and was unsure of what would be expected of me. There weren't any "back to nursing" courses at that time and I believed I would have difficulty in applying for an advertised post. So I began by approaching GOS for a part-time post, seeing as this was the hospital I was most familiar with.

By this time, Gwen Kirby had retired. I'd miss her because, although she'd been strict, she cared very much about her staff and patients. In fact, in her obituary in the 2007 *Nurses' League Journal*, an ex-staff member recalled how Matron went to visit the sickest children in the hospital every single day. Who could live up to her legacy? But I needn't have worried.

I made an appointment to see Miss Betty Barchard, the new matron, now known as chief nursing officer. The role of matron in hospitals had been re-classified as a result of the controversial Salmon Report and was beginning to be implemented from 1973. The committee behind the report had established a hierarchy from the staff nurse at Grade 5 to the chief nursing officer at Grade 10. But without a single practising nurse on the committee to lend valuable knowledge and experience, it was a disaster. It led to the demotion of ward sisters, the addition of unnecessary bureaucracy and front-line nurses becoming distanced from the lead decision maker, who was now a chief nursing officer.

Dewar wrote, "However strong the disclaimer that the Salmon committee had anything to do with salaries it was inevitable that the more highly graded administrative nurses would be paid more and the practising nurses less, and this is of course what happened.[54]

In the case of Miss Barchard, she was an experienced children's trained nurse. As a ward sister in the 1950s, she had strong convictions about children not being separated from their families and the future development of children's nursing being health promotion and care in the community. She felt that she would be able to influence this sort of change as a manager rather than as a ward sister.[55]

Consequently, she undertook an RCN management course, while working as a volunteer at GOS, and was eventually appointed their chief nursing officer.

Miss Barchard discussed the hours that I could do. I told her that John had Sunday evenings off and Monday as a day off, so I would like to work both the Sunday and Monday 12-hour night-duty shifts. I knew that eight years before, GOS had liked to employ staff they had trained themselves, but at that time, few were married. Now there were many more. What I didn't know was how many were employed part-time.

Miss Barchard knew all about me from my GOS records and was very welcoming. "I've been thinking about a new role and wondered if you might trial it for me," she said. "I'm concerned about the parents and children who turn to us for help at night. The medical staff are often too busy to see them immediately when they arrive."

Even though GOS had no accident and emergency department, this still happened. Although the children turning up were mostly known to the hospital, some weren't. The policy of never turning anyone away still remained.

"I'd like to experiment with a new role of a staff nurse assessing and referring these children to the appropriate medical team. Would you be interested?"

"Yes, I would," I said. I knew what the role would involve.

"It would also mean being on call for one or two of the hospital wards and specialling any seriously ill children if you're needed."

"I'll enjoy that, Miss Barchard," I said.

"Then the job is yours," she said. "Welcome back to GOS." And she appointed me at once.

RETURN TO GOS

I returned to GOS at the end of February 1976. Now that I was a staff nurse, I wore a red belt, and the long sleeves of my uniform were rolled up when on duty and held in place with an elasticated nylon strip known as "frills". My life had come full circle, but now I had a husband and three children. I'd had five and a half years of nursing experience and although I was out of touch, I was excited about the new challenges which faced me.

Fortunately, Philippa loved being collected from nursery and looked after by the lady across the square. Maud really spoilt her. Philippa was allowed to sit at Maud's dressing table, put on her make-up and squirt perfume from a bottle on to her neck. She'd arrive home smelling wonderful and wearing different shades of lipstick as well as powder and rouge, which, she thought, looked amazing. It did.

On my first night at GOS, I went to the night sister's office to take a hospital report from Miss Barchard. I was the only staff nurse on night duty at the time. It was still routine every evening, before the night staff arrived, for each ward sister to go to Miss Barchard's office and report on any sick child or any problems on their ward so that she could hand over to the night staff. By now the hospital had bleeps that we all carried at night. I was allocated my wards, usually two of them, and I'd visit each one at the beginning of the shift to ask some poor student to take me on a round of her patients so that I could familiarise myself with them and assess what potential problems there could be.

I was very shocked at how things had changed, particularly the new equipment on the wards. The most exciting piece of equipment was the Ivac pump, developed in the US in 1968.[56] We no longer had to count the drops of blood in the chamber every 15 minutes and rely on the roller clamp to control the amount of blood the child received – the Ivac pump did all this for us. Previously it was very laborious as it meant counting the drops while looking at our watch and regularly returning to check and alter the flow rate. Technology was developing.

The other impressive change that had taken place was the introduction of what was then known as intravenous alimentation. This was a way of giving food into a vein. It was one of the most significant advances to take place in the late 1960s. Children with bowel disorders were dying of starvation because there was no way of feeding them. Dr Stanley Dudrick, while a student at the University of Pennsylvania School of Medicine, learnt how important good nutrition was to the survival of seriously ill patients, especially during and after surgery.[57]

He had the idea of delivering concentrated nutrition to babies with bowel conditions through their veins. Controversially, he showed this could be done by successfully growing Beagle puppies (one named "Stinky") from the age of six weeks to adulthood by feeding them entirely by vein.[60]

The six puppies who were fed in this way outstripped their beagle puppy controls in weight gain and matched them in development.[58]

Subsequently in 1967, Dr Dudrick and his team applied this technique to babies born with complete obstruction to the bowel. For a year, these children grew and developed as if their guts were working normally. This marked a turning point in clinical paediatric medicine. This way of artificial feeding was now commonly being used at GOS. Because of this, and because the feed went into a child's major blood vessel, there was a risk of serious infection and blood poisoning. Replacing the feed had to be done under strict sterile conditions.[59]

As one of my back-to-work competencies, I had to be assessed changing the dressing and cleaning the area where the line entered the body, as well as changing the nutrient solution. I was overseen and marked as competent by one of the night sisters. In nursing, your training never stops. You're always learning on the job.

I enjoyed being responsible for the emergencies attending the hospital as it wasn't a role I'd performed before. I was to look after any children who arrived at the hospital with their parents. Together with the medical teams, I was responsible for receiving any children flown in at night by helicopter. When the helicopter was coming in, I was to take a large white sheet and lay it in an area of Coram Fields that was the suitable landing site, so the pilot could see where to land. I was then to assist with the transfer of the child to the hospital.

When children were brought in by their parents, I had to find the notes for any children who were already our patients. Unless the child needed urgent transfer to a ward, this was my first job. I became very efficient at tracking down these notes in the basement filing system and signing them out. I then had to inform the relevant senior house officer (SHO) and do an initial assessment before the junior doctor came to see the patient.

The child that I remember most vividly was a seven-year-old asthmatic girl who arrived with her dad. The girl was known to the hospital, having a history of respiratory infections. On initial assessment, she was very short of breath and had noisy and laboured breathing with a high pulse and respiratory rate. She had a blue tinge to her skin and I was instinctively deeply concerned about her.

I gave her some oxygen immediately and "fast bleeped" the respiratory senior house officer. (Fast bleeping was the emergency call.) Both he and the registrar were busy performing a "cut down" on a child, a surgical procedure to put a line into a vein to set up an intravenous infusion. They asked me to give the asthmatic child Ventolin to open her airways through a nebuliser using the oxygen. I took the nebuliser out of the cupboard and went to plug it in. But the plug wouldn't connect to any of the sockets in the room.

The father realised my predicament. "Let me help you," he said. "I can take the plug off one of those lights." He pointed to one of the lamps.

The girl was struggling with her breathing, so I made a quick decision. "Yes, do it, please."

"Have you got scissors?"

I handed him my blunt-ended scissors, which I always carried, and he used them to change the plug on the nebuliser. The child improved rapidly with this treatment and was managing to talk when the respiratory registrar arrived. I then found the notes and we transferred her for admission. When the day staff arrived in outpatients, I told the sister what had happened and that she now had no plug on one of her lamps. She said she would sort it.

I was on duty the next night. Before I left home, I had a phone call from Miss Barchard's secretary asking if I'd come in early to see her. I was wondering what she wanted to see me about and was reflecting on what I could have done. Miss Barchard, efficient as ever, quickly came to the point.

"I'm afraid I've had a complaint about you," she said. "The manager of the works department told me that you changed a plug on a piece of equipment last night. You must have realised that you shouldn't be tampering with electrical equipment. You should have beeped the on-call electrician if you needed a plug changed."

I explained to Miss Barchard how the child we were treating presented on arrival and how she had all signs of *status asthmaticus* (respiratory failure) in a child, which required urgent treatment. I explained, too, how the father had changed the plug and it was done extremely efficiently.

Miss Barchard didn't respond to me, but immediately contacted the works manager. She told him that the reason that I had changed this plug was that we'd had a medical emergency. She politely asked him to send his electrician first thing in the morning, as a priority to the admission room, to check that all the electrical equipment was in good working order so that this kind of incident never happened again. Miss Barchard's response was the same as Gwen

Kirby's would have been – an immediate concern for the child being admitted. I was impressed.

Then there were the children brought in who weren't our patients. Mostly, it would be a parent in an (often unnecessary) panic about their child. I would always assess and report to the relevant senior house officer on either a surgical or medical team and we would decide how to proceed. For the most part, we gave reassurance and referred the child to their GP. Occasionally, if we weren't busy, a senior house officer might stitch a small wound, or I might steri-strip it, or even lance a boil.

We had a number of children with skin rashes. I remember one child who had what looked like nettle rash on his arms and legs. On taking the history, I found that he'd been playing in the woods.

"Has he been near any nettles?" I asked his mother.

"I didn't see any," she said. "They were playing hide and seek in the bracken."

I wondered if the bracken had caused this rash. "Let me have a word with the doctor."

I phoned the senior house officer, who said to me, "I'm not sure, I'll enquire." He then phoned me back. "Yes, indeed, bracken could cause a nasty rash."

We sent the child home with antihistamine cream and advised the mother to discourage her child from playing near bracken in the future. I avoid it to this day.

While gaining this new experience of being responsible for the emergencies, Miss Barchard asked me to compile a manual to help other staff take on the role. On top of this,

I also had two wards to oversee. At 10 p.m. and 6 a.m. (and occasionally at 2 a.m.), I would go to the ward to check the medicines prescribed for the children. I would check and oversee the students giving medicines and change any intravenous lines, be on the ward to assist with emergency admissions and be bleeped if any child had problems. I would also attend any crash call with the night sisters. This was if any child had a respiratory or cardiac arrest.

As we carried bleeps by now, we and the on-call medical staff would be fast bleeped for any crash call, so that wherever we were in the hospital someone would be near to hand. Every ward and department had an arrest trolley containing all the emergency equipment and medicines that would be needed for a child of any age. These trolleys were checked daily by the ward's senior staff to make sure the equipment was in working order and to replace any medicines that had expired.

All students regularly practised resuscitation in the nursing school, and trained staff had frequent refresher courses. We would all work as a team and take on an appropriate role depending on when we arrived at the scene. Night duty was a good time for me to be able to practise my competency of resuscitation, as there were certainly nights when I remember attending calls in this large busy hospital with very sick children.

As Miss Barchard had warned me, I was also asked on some nights to special a very sick child. One was a baby with transposition of the great arteries and another was one born as a "blue baby" with a condition called Fallot's tetralogy. Both had to have emergency shunts to keep them alive, which I drew in great detail in my notebook.

I was also thrilled to have the opportunity to "special" two children with long-gap oesophageal atresia. Rachael, whom I met in outpatients in the fourth year of my training, gave me my first introduction to this condition. This helped me to have the confidence to special these children. On night duty, I would have very little support from other staff.

The first child I specialled was a newborn baby, transferred as an emergency from a local midwifery unit in an incubator. He had a special tube, called a Replogle tube, through his nose to keep his airway clear of spit. This tube was on continuous suction and needed consistent monitoring and flushing to keep it clear. It was a temporary measure to keep the child alive before his first surgical operation.

The second child was older. He'd already had his first operations – closing his fistula and creating an opening on his neck for "sham feeding". I was specialling him following his final operation to restore his anatomy. Surgery had progressed to an operation called the Heimlich operation. Henry Heimlich was a heart surgeon who is famous for inventing the Heimlich manoeuvre, which has saved thousands of people from choking to death. This is a form of bear hug to apply abdominal thrusts from behind on someone who's choking. In America, this choking was often referred to as Beefsteak Disease since among adults it usually involved swallowing large bites of meat that hadn't been thoroughly chewed, but the risk to children ingesting foreign objects was just as severe.[60]

The child that I specialled following the Heimlich's operation had a long section of the stomach shaped into a tube. This tube was inverted and pulled up to replace the oesophagus. I drew a picture of this operation in my notebook at the time.

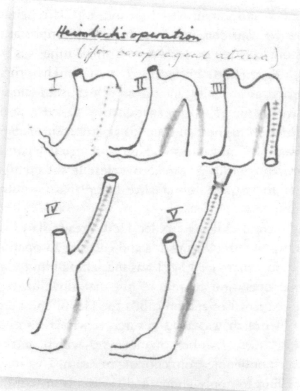

A page from my notebook from night duty in 1976.

The advantages of this operation over the one to transplant a piece of bowel were that it could be performed without the surgeon having to open the child's chest cavity and the newly grafted area had a much better blood supply. Both meant that recovery from surgery was quicker, and feeding by mouth could start sooner.

Because part of the operation took place in the neck area, and swelling could occur (which might affect breathing), I nursed the child on an Engström ventilator, which were still in use and very familiar to me. Children tended to swallow air after the operation and it was important that their stomach didn't swell up, so a small tube was passed through their nose and into their stomach. The other end of the tube was attached to an underwater seal drain by the bed, through which any air would pass. I enjoyed caring for both of these children and was glad that I had met Rachael 10 years before.

Specialling children at night was an ideal time to learn about all these conditions and gain experience in intensive care nursing. What I was unable to do when specialling and on night duty was to have any relationship with the child or the family and to follow up the child after their treatment. I did feel the absence of this connection, and despite the fast-paced lifestyle in emergency care, I wished I could still have strong bonds with the individual children.

Another of my experiences was specialling a young boy who was one of a pair of conjoined twins. They were born joined from the chest to the abdomen and facing each other. Though they had separate hearts, they shared many of their other organs. The liver, in particular, caused huge complications. The operation to separate them took 12 hours, and five surgeons were involved.

The children were nursed together in 1A's pump room, which was big enough to take both children. Another staff nurse and I specialled one child each for two nights. The liver had been divided during surgery and was bleeding badly. According to Professor Spitz, who is world-renowned for leading surgical teams in the separation of conjoined twins, the successful separation of the liver requires great skill. These days, surgical teams use an ultrasound dissector, which vibrates at an extraordinary high rate and shakes the liver cells to pieces. Those pieces are extracted so that the blood vessels can be sealed and divided.[61] This wasn't an option at that time.

By the second night, the twins were still bleeding. We tried to replace the blood lost as best we could, but at some point during the shift, the blood pressure of the child I was looking after began to drop. I had to syringe the blood into the venous line to try to maintain his blood pressure at a reasonable level. We had no break in our 12-hour night shift, were constantly being fed chocolate milk shakes through straws and were exhausted by the end of it.

Unfortunately, these twins did not survive. The boys had been through so much in their short lives, and it was painful to think of all the things they would never experience. As a mother myself, I could understand these parents' anguish now that their worst fears had become fact.

As I left the hospital, a passer-by asked me if I knew anything about the twins and I had to deny all knowledge of them. We were sworn to secrecy over any patients, especially high-profile ones. We often watched vulturous reporters sneaking up the hospital drive when there was something interesting going on, trying to get a picture or to accost some poor tired nurse leaving the hospital.

Conjoined twins are extremely rare – only one in every 2.5 million births. In 2019, Great Ormond Street Hospital, now identified as GOSH, successfully separated sisters Safa and Marwa Ullah. The two-year-olds from Pakistan, born by caesarean section, were craniopagus twins (fused at the head) – an incredibly rare condition. They needed three major operations and a number of small procedures.

GOSH experts used cutting-edge technology, such as virtual reality and 3D printing, to decide the best strategy and optimise the chances of success. An exact replica of the girls' anatomy was created in virtual reality to help the surgeons visualise and understand their complex skulls and spatial relation between their brains and blood vessels. To make the operations as effective as possible, 3D plastic models of their brains, skulls and blood vessels were then printed. The surgeons could practise the surgery and build cutting guides on these replicas.[62] As well as using this technology on these two girls, the same team at GOSH successfully separated twin boys from Turkey who were joined at the head, in January 2020.

In January 1977, there must have been a flu epidemic as night sisters started dropping like flies. In three months, I'd gone from covering two hospital wards at night to six wards. It was hectic and I rarely had a break. I was doing more than a night sister's role as I was covering emergencies as well.

After Easter, I made an appointment to see Miss Barchard. She was pleased to see me and asked me how I was getting on in her new role in the admissions area. She thanked me for compiling the manual to help other staff in the role and said how useful it would be. I then reminded her about the sickness rate of night sisters and how I was now overseeing up to six wards in the hospital as well as assessing any emergencies arriving unannounced.

"I wondered if you'd consider giving me a night sister's post if I increased my nights to three, which would be to 36 hours a week."

Miss Barchard looked at me, considering my proposal. I knew it was a long shot but if you don't ask, you don't get.

"I really do appreciate how hard you're working, covering for staff sickness . . ." she said.

I nodded but knew there was a "but" coming.

". . . But policy is only to appoint sisters on a full-time basis, which would be 48 hours per week. Would that be possible for you?"

I knew this would never work for our family life, which was hectic enough as it was.

"I'm sorry, Miss Barchard, but I couldn't manage that with three children."

Later, I discussed this conversation with John. Always ready for a challenge, he began to buy nursing journals to see if any part-time night sister's posts were being advertised in other hospitals. We found three suitable advertisements in paediatrics, all within commuting distance from our home. One was at St George's Hospital, the second was at Lewisham Hospital and the third was at Brompton Hospital. I applied for all three. I was sent letters from each hospital inviting me for interview and was offered all three posts.

I chose to accept the post at Brompton Hospital as Miss Muirhead, the much-respected matron, offered me my preferred three nights in a row – Sunday, Monday and Tuesday. The other hospitals couldn't guarantee consecutive nights. However, I was flattered to receive a letter from St George's saying that they were sorry I was unable to accept their post of part-time night sister, adding: "Should you ever wish to apply to St George's Hospital in the future we will be extremely happy to consider your application."

Once again, I arranged to see Miss Barchard to tell her that I would be handing in my notice as I had been offered a night sister's post for three nights a week at Brompton Hospital. She said how sorry she was to lose me from her staff and wished me well.

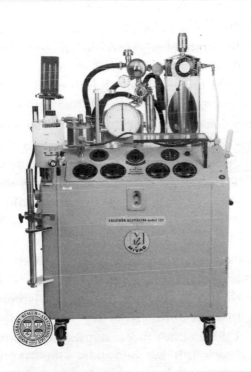

The iconic Engström Ventilator.

ROYAL BROMPTON
HOSPITAL

Royal Brompton Hospital, situated in Chelsea, is the largest specialist heart and lung centre in the UK. Known as Brompton Hospital when I worked there, it was granted a Royal Charter by Queen Elizabeth II in 1991.

It had an interesting beginning. It was built in 1841 and was the only hospital in England and Wales that would take patients with tuberculosis (TB). There was no cure for tuberculosis, or consumption as it was called at the time. It was highly infectious and was described as the "white plague". It was the world's top infectious killer before Covid-19.[63] Although tuberculosis is spread by bacterial infection, not a virus, it has many parallels to Covid-19 and is deadly in its effects. It's been largely controlled in the UK by compulsory vaccination.

Solicitor Philip Rose built Brompton Hospital after discovering that one of his clerks had tuberculosis and was appalled to find that he'd been refused admission to any hospital in London. It was originally called the Hospital for Consumption and Diseases of the Chest. Like GOS, it depended on the kindness of benefactors. Many, including

Queen Victoria, who became their patron, gave them an annual donation of £10.

In 1871, the then Brompton Hospital was left a huge legacy of nearly £100,000 from a Miss Read, an eccentric lady who lived in squalor and collected pieces of string and paper bags. Distant relatives failed to overturn her will after paying for a post-mortem to try to prove that she had brain disease and wasn't of sound mind. This donation enabled the hospital to double its bed capacity.

The hospital was renowned for its research and innovation. It produced the Brompton cough lozenges in 1886, which were sold on stalls on the Fulham Road for a penny a box, and the Brompton Cocktail, a mixture of morphine, cocaine, alcohol and chloroform, given in the distressing terminal stages of tuberculosis.[64]

In July 1977, I started as a night sister on the 22-bed children's ward called Rose Gallery, named after the hospital's founder, Philip Rose. My three nights away from home meant that life was more hectic for John. We had to make sure our routine was carefully organised. It meant that three mornings a week, he had to get the children up, dressed and breakfasted and ready for school as I didn't return home until about 9 a.m.

To make matters worse, each child now went to a different school. Jonathan was still collected and brought home from the Sybil Elgar School for autistic children in Ealing. James, now six, was attending St James' Primary School, and Philippa, now four, was at Kintore Way Nursery. The last two were local but in different directions.

Fortunately, Maud was very happy to take Philippa three mornings a week to Kintore Way, then collect her and give her tea afterwards. Philippa was thrilled to have Maud to herself for an extra afternoon and to be a bit more independent from the boys.

As I slept until 3 p.m. on Mondays and Tuesdays, I could collect James from school every afternoon and make the evening meal for the family. John had a day off on Monday but had to make sure that any meetings he had were held at the vicarage on Tuesday evenings so that he was in the house with the children. He was now responsible for putting the children to bed three nights a week, not two. James and Philippa were easy to settle at night, but Jonathan was still very active, not settling until the early hours of the morning. It was amazing how the other two slept while Jonathan rushed around.

Jonathan was now nine and Professor Robinson was still seeing him regularly at Guy's Hospital. In my early days at Brompton Hospital, Professor Robinson asked us if we'd like Jonathan to be assessed by Professor Rutter at Maudsley Hospital. The Professor was an expert in autism. We agreed and took Jonathan to the Maudsley one day for an outpatient appointment. We weren't included in his assessment, but we gathered that Jonathan would be left to play in an area with special toys while being observed by Professor Rutter and his specialist team. Meanwhile, we sat in the waiting room for almost an hour before being called into the consulting room. Here Professor Rutter introduced us to his team and then told us his verdict, very bluntly.

"We have diagnosed Jonathan with autism," he said.

I burst into tears, even though I knew it was a possibility.

"This woman needs help," Professor Rutter said. Then he turned to his child psychologist. "Make an appointment to see Mrs Martin."

The meeting was over and we were sent home.

The following week, I was visited at home by the child psychologist. We worked out that my biggest problem at that time was Jonathan's lack of sleep, and hence mine and John's. He still only slept for four and a half hours a night and consistently left his room to come downstairs, as by now he could easily dismantle any gate we erected in his doorway.

The psychologist designed a large dinosaur calendar with dates on it, for me to make and hang on the wall outside the living room. I was to reward Jonathan with a star to put on the date of every night that he didn't come out of his bedroom. I duly made this dinosaur calendar, bought large stars to stick on it and told Jonathan what we were going to do. On the odd night that he didn't leave his room, I made a big celebration of sticking a star on the calendar. Jonathan showed no interest in it at all. It gave him no encouragement to stay in his room.

Professor Rutter and the child psychologist never saw us again.

I continued to cycle to and from work. The journey to Brompton Hospital was going to take me longer as it was six miles from my home instead of the 4.4 miles to GOS. Before I started on my new ward, I had to be measured for my uniform. The measurements taken were far more exact than those at GOS. As a result, the uniforms were a beautiful fit and very comfortable. I also had my usual health check, which included having a Heaf test (now the Mantoux test is used instead). This was a skin test to check if I had resistance to tuberculosis. As this test showed that my antibody resistance was low, it was recommended that I should have a second BCG vaccination. I arrived to have my vaccination and was approached by one of the respiratory consultants.

He told me that he was about to give a lecture to medical students on tuberculosis. "Would you mind awfully if I gave you your BCG vaccination?" I was surprised as I wasn't expecting it to be given by one of the medical staff, let alone the consultant. "I'd like to give it in the lecture theatre. I'd like to demonstrate on you to show these students how it should be done."

"I suppose it's better than demonstrating on an orange."

"Indeed it is, Sister."

So it was agreed.

I was taken into the amphitheatre of the hospital education department, which was full of male medical students, and then, as requested, I stripped to my bra to have this injection. After a talk on the testing for tuberculosis, the vaccine and the treatments, which took some time, I was finally given the vaccination, thanked for my help and allowed to leave. I do wonder how much my half-nakedness distracted the medical students from the talk! It was definitely an unusual introduction to my new appointment.

Each evening I would approach the hospital for my night shift along a tunnel to the south side entrance. There were many notices in the tunnel, saying "This is a Chest Hospital. To Protect Our Patients, Please Do Not Smoke". It was the first hospital I'd come across where I saw no one smoking, even in the hospital grounds.

On Rose Gallery, I was responsible for children with chest and heart conditions. The medical and surgical children were nursed in separate bays. We also had a four-bedded high dependency bay on the ward, where we would special children who'd undergone open heart surgery and were not ventilated.

The hospital had a number of postgraduate students who were working to gain a qualification in chest and heart disease. Many came from the Far East and were working with me and the staff nurses on the ward. I had up to four of these students as well as a staff nurse as part of my team. The postgraduate students, having gained registered nurse certificates in their own country, were able to special in the high dependency bay. They were overseen by me and the staff nurse. They also assisted in the main ward area.

Many children with heart problems came to the hospital from Saudi Arabia, paid for by the Saudi government. Their mothers would be resident on the ward as we had folding beds so that parents could sleep by their child. They would help us to prepare their child for theatre in the early morning, as children would always be first on the operating lists. Although interpreters were available during the day, we had none at night, which could lead to some impromptu charades on both sides. The normal routine was that the child would be bathed, dressed in a hospital gown for easy access to the operation site and given the usual injection of a sedative and a medicine to dry the saliva in their mouth. This premedication injection would be given at least an hour before the operation started.

The problem with some of the mothers from Saudi Arabia is that not all of them would undress their children to put them to bed, let alone undress them for theatre. Some were constantly dressed in their day clothes. Discussing this with a Pakistani friend of mine, she told me that this wouldn't have been anything to do with Islam. It was likely to do with fear and a complete lack of understanding of our culture and what happens to people in our hospitals. I would sit and try to talk to these mothers, which wasn't easy without an interpreter, indicating that they could undress, bath and put their child in the gown themselves. Some would eventually agree to do this for me. A small minority would refuse adamantly.

Much to the frustration of the theatre staff, we would have to take these children to the anaesthetic room in their own clothes, where they would be anaesthetised, undressed, washed and put into a gown before being allowed into the theatre. This would delay the list for at least 20 minutes. Interestingly enough, these parents would never refuse the injection of premedication for their child, perhaps because I made it clear that it was to help them sleep.

I always checked the prescriptions and prepared the premedication equipment well before the time due. I then rechecked them with the staff nurse or student when it was the time to give them. Children's doses are prescribed by the weight of the child, whereas for adults there's a recommended dose. It was always important to check and recheck the doses prescribed for the injections before drawing them up in the syringe at the appropriate times.

One morning, I was checking and preparing these

injections for the cardiac list when I noticed an error of one decimal point in one of the baby's prescriptions due at 7 a.m. It was now 6.30. I bleeped the anaesthetist who had prescribed the medicine. He was furious, demanding to know what was important enough for me to wake him at that hour. I told him what he had prescribed for the baby's premedication, gave him the weight of the child and said that I realised he would not like me to give the child 10 times the recommended dose. He calmed down. I asked him if he would like to re-write the prescription himself. Otherwise I was quite prepared to change it, give the medicine and sign the prescription if he would come to the ward before theatre and countersign my alteration. He said that I could alter the prescription and he would sign it before I went off duty. He arrived on the ward at about 7.15 to sign the prescription. He apologised for the way he had spoken to me on the phone, saying he was very grateful that I had contacted him.

I met this anaesthetist at other times in the hospital and we often chatted. He asked me one day if I'd been to watch any of the open-heart surgery on our children. When I said I hadn't, he introduced me to the teaching theatre with a viewing room. It was an amazing facility that I'd never seen before.

I stayed on after my shift one morning. I was in an enclosed gallery of mostly glass, overlooking the theatre table where certain operations could be viewed and teaching took place without having to go into the theatre itself. I could stand and watch the operation while listening to the surgeon's commentary on what he was doing. I watched a child of ours having his vessels attached to the heart-lung machine and saw the heart stop beating so the operation could take place. I watched the operation, then the vessels being taken off the by-pass machine and reconnected to the heart, which started working normally again. It was fascinating and well worth giving up some sleep to watch.

While I was on Rose Gallery, I nursed a lovely child called Eric. He was eight years old and had had a hole in the heart since birth. The hole was between the two lower chambers of his heart, called the ventricles. This is the most common heart defect. Eric had been followed up by the heart physicians since he was a baby and had had a major operation in the past. A patch of synthetic material called Dacron was sewn over the hole while his heart was connected to the heart-lung machine. He was on the ward being reviewed by the physicians and having tests. One test involved injecting a dye into a vein leading to his heart. X-ray images could be taken of his heart so the physician could see what might be causing his mild heart failure.

Eric was lively and chatty and would often come and sit with me if he couldn't settle to sleep and I wasn't too busy. He had a favourite toy that he brought into hospital with him. His mother often stayed with him at night, so I got to know her too. Eric's biggest problem was the cocktail of medicines that he had to take regularly. It included digoxin (to steady his heartbeat), an antibiotic, two more tablets known as water tablets, and finally potassium. He *hated* them. His mother and I had to give him lots of praise and the occasional treat to encourage him to swallow them. During his stay in hospital, the medical staff were trying to reduce the number of his medicines, while monitoring the effect on his heart.

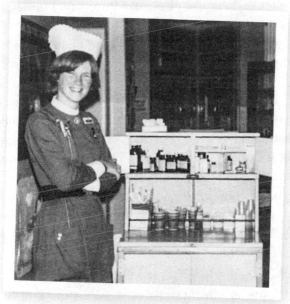

Me with the drug trolley, which Eric hated!

After Eric was discharged home, he wrote me a long letter. He told me that he was being good and taking all his medicines now that he wasn't having such a cocktail of them all. He thanked me for all I had done to make him well again and asked me to give his best wishes to the other sisters on the ward. He told me about his visit to his local hospital, where a registrar had taken a sample of his blood to examine the electrolytes (blood minerals). Eric wrote in his letter:

"Doctor Scott took some blood for my electric lights and they were negative, so they have cut down my medicines."

223

He added: "I have a teacher coming to the house now and she is very nice."

He enclosed a recent photo of himself, on holiday, saying: "This is so you can see how well I look now."

Eric wasn't admitted again to Rose Gallery while I was there, but I heard from him again the following year. He wrote:

"Dear Vanessa,

I am sorry I haven't written to you, as I have been very busy and working hard at school, as I would very much like to go to university. We have moved recently. The doctors at the hospital said I am getting on very well, and now I have started horse riding."

Eric then asked me if I would send him a photo of my husband and family, which I did. After that, we lost touch.

Royal Marsden Hospital was situated across the road from Brompton Hospital. Its canteen on the ground floor was open at night, and this was where the Brompton staff were invited for their meals. For the first month, I tried the canteen and enjoyed meeting some of the Royal Marsden staff. I then realised that the other staff brought sandwiches and ate them on Rose Gallery. As one of my roles was teaching, it seemed an ideal opportunity to teach the postgraduate students during their meal break and they were keen for me to do this. I set up a teaching package, which included explanations and illustrations of congenital (present at birth) heart conditions, and began to teach them in small groups.

It appeared to be a success. I enjoyed this teaching opportunity as it kept me more up-to-date with the

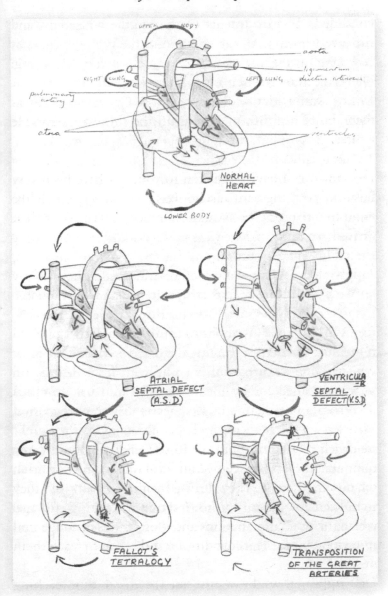

Here's an illustration I made of heart conditions.

conditions and treatments of the children I cared for. I, too, was learning. All the children in the high-dependency bay were on cardiac monitors, which are very popular in television dramas when a character is admitted to hospital. I had to know and be able to recognise all of the different rhythms of the heart and how they should be treated.

One busy night, the high-dependency bay was full. At 2 a.m. a child had a cardiac arrest in the bay. The heart monitor was showing the dreaded straight line. I was very familiar with the ward arrest trolley as I checked all the equipment and the medicines every night. The arrest team arrived promptly, and we were in the middle of resuscitating the child when a second child arrested. I took charge of supplying the relevant instruments and medicines.

We had just one anaesthetist, who had already intubated the first child (put a tube into his throat to help get oxygen to his lungs) and was about to intubate the second child. I remember hurriedly changing the blade on that instrument while having to throw other equipment from bed to bed as it was called for by medical staff. I also had to check and draw up medicines in syringes as they were requested. This was all done surprisingly calmly by us as a team. We managed to stabilise both children, who were then taken temporarily back to the adult intensive care unit from where they'd come. They survived with no ill effects, much to our delight. Later I was to find out that the hospital had created a paediatric intensive care unit, which was a real improvement for children and for their care.

One morning, while waiting for the day staff to arrive, I was with a group of children and we were looking out of the ward window at the view. Suddenly, the body of a man flashed past the window.

One child shouted: "Was that a man?"

I quickly replied that I thought it was just something that had fallen from the roof and guided them all towards the playroom, where the nursery nurse had arrived and was setting out toys. Luckily, the children were quickly distracted. All the hospital ward windows had bars on them, so I knew the man who had jumped had come from the roof. How he got there, I never learnt. As I was at the end of my stretch of three nights, I never found out any more about him.

As heartbreaking as it always was, it wasn't unusual for the occasional patient to commit suicide in this hospital as many of the cardiac patients had life-threatening conditions. I was confident the incident would have been thoroughly investigated by Miss Muirhead.

Miss Muirhead was a shy but efficient matron. I would often meet her when the hospital was short-staffed and I was asked to be on call for emergencies and to help out with checking controlled medicines on some of the adult wards. I would then go to her office to hand over any problems that the wards had experienced during the night.

One particular event has a nasty resonance now as such terrible information has since emerged. An evening drinks and buffet party had been arranged for all the nurses in the hospital. This was an invitation to meet the guest of honour who had funded the event, Jimmy Savile. I had been to one of these events before at GOS and don't remember enjoying it much, but I was persuaded to go by the ward staff. I went with John as we were allowed to bring a partner. What I remember about this event was Jimmy Savile grabbing poor

Miss Muirhead's arm and sitting her on his knee. We could all see how uncomfortable she was and, although a few in the room laughed, I think most of us were embarrassed for her. John and I decided not to stay.

John's father was approaching retirement from his parish in Betchworth, Surrey, which would mean his parents were moving out of their vicarage. They would need a home. If they sold their life insurance policy, their entire life savings came to £2,000, enough to buy them a small croft in the North of Scotland. John's income was £1,000 a year and we could get a mortgage of three and a half times that. So we came to the decision that we and John's parents would buy a cottage together. Our hope was that, when they were in their 90s and we ourselves came to retire, they would be happy for us to join them!

We looked at Cambridgeshire, which was as near to London as we could afford. We found a cottage in Outwell, in the diocese of Ely, and John was offered two parishes there. Although he'd loved working in Bermondsey for nine years, he was ready to meet and work with a whole new range of people. It was 1978 – Jonathan was 10, James seven and a half and Philippa was five.

I told Miss Muirhead immediately and gave her three months' notice of my leaving. She said that she would be sorry to see me go, which I appreciated as I'd enjoyed working at the Brompton so much. Miss Muirhead called me to her office two weeks later and said that she had advertised my post and had appointed a replacement night sister for Rose Gallery. She then asked me if I would like to deputise for the night nursing officer for my last two months. It would mean my working on the general side. It also meant that I would be in charge of the hospital when the night nursing officer was on her nights off. I said I would enjoy the experience very much.

I began working mostly on the adult side. I would only be on call for Rose Gallery if there was a problem. I would take the handover report from Miss Muirhead in her office. It would include very ill patients, incidents that had taken place, and any staffing problems. It wasn't the tradition at the Brompton to go around the wards asking for a report on the patients, because at night the wards were run by a staff nurse and qualified adult-trained nurses doing postgraduate training. I did, though, have to check each ward's controlled medicines. I also attended cardiac arrests, helped out with emergency admissions and took enquiries from the press. The night staff nurses would bleep me if they needed my help in any way. I soon got to know some of the patients and many of the staff in the hospital that I had never had contact with before.

We had many emergency admissions during the night, particularly medical emergencies with chest problems. On one of my shifts, a lady in her late 40s was admitted having a severe asthmatic attack. I was fast bleeped to attend her cardiac arrest call, but tragically she died. The staff were very upset. She was from Scotland and had been visiting friends in London. I took all her details and prepared myself for what I knew would be a difficult experience.

It was the first phone call like this that I'd had to make to a family. Near the end of my shift, I spoke to the husband. He had extended family living with him at the time, helping him through this difficult time. He was obviously destroyed by the news of his wife's death.

"Will you wait on the line please, Sister," he whispered, "while I tell the rest of the family."

"Of course I will," I said.

I waited for a while and I could hear talking and crying. It was heartbreaking. Then he came back on the line and asked for the address of the hospital and whom to contact. He and her parents planned to come over that day and arrange for his wife's body to be collected. This must have been the most difficult journey they'd ever had to take.

In the morning at the end of my shift, I gave my handover report to Miss Muirhead and she thanked me for the trouble I had taken with the family. I often had a lot to tell her at our morning handover meetings and she once commented:

"More seems to happen when you are on duty, Sister Martin."

I don't know if that was true but there were certainly moments of drama.

One thing about working as a nurse is that you never know what's going to happen. Every shift is different and gives staff opportunities to learn. One of my more rewarding experiences at the Brompton was working with patients with cystic fibrosis. They were now living into their late teens because their care had improved so much. Patients from GOS were being transferred here to be looked after by the respiratory team as soon as they reached the age of 16 and were classed as adults.

This team had established the first adult cystic fibrosis clinic in 1965 and helped to make the hospital the largest treatment and research centre for these patients in Europe.

They were taking their knowledge and expertise into other communities by running joint clinics in local district general hospitals.[64] I was able to help with some of the care of these patients, particularly with their physiotherapy.

I'd seen my physiotherapist mother treat patients and she had shown me how to "tip and clap". Patients would lie over a foam mattress with their head hung down. Then with cupped hands I would clap the sides of their chest to loosen their congestion and clear their phlegm. It was something that I could teach other staff to do. When I was free to do so, I regularly went round the medical wards and helped staff give care to these patients.

I was sorry to leave Brompton Hospital. I'd learnt an incredible amount in my short time working there. I was anxious about leaving London, convinced that any experience outside the capital would be far less stimulating. How wrong I was.

NORTH CAMBRIDGESHIRE HOSPITAL

We moved into the old vicarage on the west side of St George's, the main parish church of Littleport in Cambridgeshire. A new vicarage was to be built in the old vicarage's paddock, but for now we were living in a vast old house. Upstairs, there were seven bedrooms (two of which had been servants' rooms), two dressing rooms and two bathrooms. Downstairs, there was a large hall with an impressive staircase and, to the left of the hall, was John's study. To the right, there was a huge room, so large that it had been used in the past for bible classes for as many as 100 men. The church crèche was held in there during services. Behind this room was a dining room which we never used.

Because the central heating was old and too expensive to run, the parlour became our family room as it was the warmest in the house. Philippa (aged five) would be washed in a metal bath here in the winter before being carried up the back stairs to her bed, which had been warmed with a hot water bottle. John used to answer the telephone in his study in his coat. He'd sit at his desk shivering in the draught that blew through the gaps in the window frames that were large enough to put a hand through.

The vicarage grounds were also large. As well as the paddock, there was an orchard and a separate coach house and stables. The latter were used to store wastepaper, collected by parishioners, which was then sold by the ton to raise funds for the church.

Philippa and James went to the local primary school opposite the church. Jonathan was still at Sybil Elgar School in London but was a weekly boarder, as we wanted him at home as much as possible. Either John or I took him to London by train from Littleport station on a Monday and collected him on a Friday.

One morning, John was dropping Jonathan and me off at the station in the car to get the 6.30 train. He returned to the vicarage to find two worried children in the hallway with big eyes. John had been gone for 10 minutes.

"Daddy," said James, "I've just phoned the police and told them we were alone in the house and didn't know where you were. They're sending a policeman to come and see us."

"My Godfathers," said John and began to look up the Ely police station telephone number. He thought the police were relieved that the second phone call came through so quickly, but they said they'd already dispatched a policewoman who would be with us shortly.

The policewoman arrived and came into the vicarage. She spoke to the children. "Are you James?" she asked.

He said he was.

Then she asked: "Are you Philippa?"

She said she was.

Reassured that the children were well, she turned to John for an explanation. He told her all about Jonathan and that he'd only been gone for 10 minutes. She said that John ought not really to leave the children, even for a short while. John made a mental note to tell the children the night before when he had to drive Jonathan and me to the station.

St George's was an impressive church with a sixteenth-century tower housing a peel of eight bells to call people to church. They were loved by wedding couples. Later, Philippa would be part of the team that rang the bells. John remembers standing on the top of the tower as an anti-tank plane from either Lakenheath or Mildenhall flew over our new vicarage. John was slightly above the pilot, looking down on him.

The church was very popular for weddings, with John taking up to three every Saturday in the summer. Before we had the improvements to the church, wedding guests would just walk into the vicarage asking to use the toilet or looking for the rubbish bin. We felt very much that we were living in a public space.

When we came to Littleport, John was licensed to the parishes as "Priest-in-Charge". This was because the diocese wanted to sell the old vicarage and build a new one in the paddock and, if John had been instituted as vicar, he could have refused to move. No one could have insisted. So the Bishop licensed him at a special service that Jonathan, James and Philippa and I attended. John was only 36, and the youngest clergyman in the Ely area at that time.

But there was a problem with this. On our arrival at Littleport, some people believed that, because John was licensed to the parish and not the vicar, he was only there temporarily. This meant that they didn't take him seriously and it was harder for him to do his job. So, John went to the

Bishop and told him his dilemma. They agreed that John would move vicarages – we actually didn't wish to stay with our family in that vast cold house – and the Bishop would institute him as vicar.

The institution service took place 18 months after our arrival, and Jonathan attended with me and the family. In the middle of the service, Jonathan threw a tantrum. John's parents, who were with us, insisted on taking him out and walking him round the church grounds until the service finished.

That night, John and I went up to his room.

John asked the question we sometimes asked. "Why were you angry, Jonathan?"

"I don't want to move," Jonathan said.

We were both surprised. This was the first time Jonathan had ever told us why he'd had a tantrum. We realised that the licensing and the institution services were very similar to each other, so Jonathan had associated them with our family moving.

"Don't worry, Jonathan," John said. "We're not moving this time."

We felt that we'd made a communication breakthrough. It was another 18 months before the new vicarage in the paddock was ready and, by then, Jonathan knew where his room would be and was happy to move in.

What we did begin to notice was that although Sybil Elgar School was good for Jonathan academically, he was losing his ability to talk to people. When we collected him from school on a Friday, John and I both remarked how our son and his fellow pupils sat around in silence, not talking to each other. The only communication seemed to come from the teachers. This was so different to Jonathan's primary school in Bermondsey where his fellow pupils had chatted to him constantly.

It was time to look for a nursing job. I applied for a part-time paediatric ward sister's post at North Cambridgeshire Hospital, a manageable three-quarters of an hour drive from home. The post was for four days a week, and I was very pleased to be accepted at the interview. This would be my first ward sister's post.

North Cambridgeshire Hospital was a small general hospital in the centre of Wisbech. It had a medical unit, a surgical unit, a children's ward, theatres, laboratories and an accident and emergency department, open from 9 a.m. to 5 p.m. Clarkson Hospital, a geriatric and respite hospital, was on a nearby site and the two hospitals were managed together. Both hospitals were efficiently run, and everyone knew each other. The newly built Queen Elizabeth Hospital in King's Lynn, about 15 miles away, was a teaching hospital and sent nursing students to Wisbech for experience. The nursing school was training students to become state registered nurses (a three-year training) and were also doing state enrolled nurses training (a two-year training to become "practical nurses"). These nurses would come to the ward for their three-month children's experience and I would be responsible for their teaching. I was required to be assessed by the School of Nursing on my competency to examine students in a practical setting. My assessment to become a student nurse examiner took place in June that year.

When I was introduced to the staff on the ward, I met Senior Staff Nurse Duffy, an Irish lady who had been acting up as ward sister since the previous sister retired after 30 years' service. At first, I was nervous about how she'd respond to having a new ward sister, but I needn't have worried. Staff Nurse Duffy welcomed me with open arms.

"We've never had a sick children's trained nurse as part of our team before," she said. "It's really exciting."

Within a few days, everyone in the hospital appeared to know I'd trained at Great Ormond Street Children's Hospital.

The first thing I noticed after my appointment was that the ward had no paediatric resuscitation equipment. Jubilee Ward admitted children from babies upwards with a wide range of medical conditions, burns injuries, orthopaedic conditions and those requiring ENT surgery. Sick children can deteriorate very quickly, therefore it's essential to have all the necessary equipment to hand to resuscitate them.

Staff Nurse Duffy was delighted to help me set up a suitable resuscitation trolley. She liaised with the paediatric anaesthetist who provided me with all the appropriate sizes of equipment and the medicines that might be needed. I made sure that the night staff checked the trolley regularly, not only to familiarise themselves with what was on it, but to make sure that the medicines remained in date. I also found that the equipment for taking blood pressures only had an adult cuff. Even though younger children don't often have their blood pressure taken, I believed it was important to cater for all, so Staff Nurse Duffy helped me order appropriately sized cuffs to fit every age group.

My contract stated that I, along with the two other sisters who ran the adult wards, was expected to act as the senior nursing officer, Miss Bradder, on a regular basis in her absence. This would mean being in charge of the hospital. To be able to do this, I would have to work the occasional night duty shift.

One of the paediatric anaesthetists asked me if I'd ever had the opportunity to take samples of blood from children or to intubate them (put a tube in their throat to help their lungs expand). When I said I hadn't, he invited me to work with him in theatre. Under his supervision, I took blood, I put tubes into veins to give patients intravenous fluids and I intubated patients of various ages. It was a good learning experience. In the future, when nursing practice changed, we nurses had to take on extended roles. Taking blood and putting tubes into veins became common practice.

There was never any time to sit around on Jubilee Ward. We had regular ENT operating lists for children needing their tonsils and adenoids removed or the insertion of grommets – a small tube used to ventilate the middle ear. We had some orthopaedic children on traction, moved from Queen Elizabeth Hospital so that they could recover nearer their families. We had medical children, mostly with respiratory problems, who required steam inhalations or regular nebulisers. We also admitted many burns patients from A&E, just as I had experienced at Queen Mary's Hospital Roehampton, with burns from fires or, more frequently, from grabbing the handle of a boiling pan from a stove. Any major burns were sent to Norfolk and Norwich Hospital, which had a specialist unit, but more minor burns were treated in Wisbech.

Mr Thompson, our burns and plastics consultant, told me about a new technique of using pressure garments on burns patients to try to prevent the unsightly scars that some of them had to suffer. Together, we decided to experiment on two boys with similar burns that were suitable for the wearing of these made-to-measure elasticated garments.

The first child, Ian, was only two years old. He was admitted to our ward from A&E with an extremely painful burn to his right arm. The family lived in a caravan on a site in Wisbech. On the evening that Ian was admitted, his mum had been deep-frying chips for the family's supper. Ian had grabbed the handle of the chip pan on the stove, pouring boiling fat over his right arm. The treatment of the child's shock was the first priority. Ian was sedated and given strong painkillers in A&E. The calculation of the burns area was made and an intravenous infusion set up. He was then transferred to Jubilee Ward into our care.

When he arrived, I cleaned and dressed Ian's wounds along with one of the staff nurses. He then slept peacefully and the staff nurse specialled him. My next priority was to look after his mum. She, too, was very shocked and upset. I remember making her a cup of tea and reassuring her that this was not her fault and that Ian would make a good recovery.

Ian's wounds were slow to heal, so Mr Thompson took Ian to the operating theatre for extensive cleaning and removal of dead tissue from the wounds. When it *had* healed, I measured John for three elastic vests that he would have to wear, with a long sleeve that would put pressure on the scarred area of his right arm. He would have to wear these vests continuously for a year, only taking them off for washing. He and his mum had an appointment to see me every first Monday of the month to check they were coping with the garments and to have his scars recorded by the hospital photographer.

I found that the vests irritated him at night, and although applying creams to his skin helped, Mr Thomson and I decided to abandon the vests and have Ian fitted for a single-arm garment with body straps. This was much more successful and easier for his mum to manage. The garments were meant to be worn until his scarred areas were no longer red or active. After 15 months, the scars on Ian's arm looked white and he could stop wearing his garment, much to his mum's relief.

The second child to wear a pressure garment, Alan, was one year and eight months old. He was visiting his grandmother when he grabbed the tea cosy over a newly made pot of tea, spilling the tea over his chest and right arm. His burn area was more extensive than Ian's and once he recovered from the initial burn, he also had to have accurate measurements made for an elastic vest. This time, the pressure was to be concentrated on his chest area as well as his right arm. Alan also experienced skin irritation from the garment, but not as much as Ian. Baby lotion applied regularly to his skin appeared to relieve this. We did need to have the vests made longer, down to his naval, as he had a little pot belly and they kept riding up. It was 18 months before Alan's scars were white and I discussed removing the vests with Alan's mum. She wanted to wait until the weather was warmer, and after discussing it with her, I agreed. So Alan wore them for a further three months.

What interested Mr Thompson was that when Alan began to wear these garments, he had noticed a contracted scar in his armpit. He thought this would stop him extending his arm and he would have to operate on it at a later date. Usually, these areas of scarring become tighter and harder as the scar heals. However, we noticed that with the wearing of these garments, this area became softer and more supple, and the extension of Alan's arm improved. We felt that these garments could benefit patients cosmetically, but also reduce both raised and contracting scars. We proposed to continue their use.

Throughout the treatment of both boys, the hospital photographer had photographed the scars as they healed so that we could see how they progressed using the garments. I wrote up this research. It was accepted for publication and was published in the *Nursing Mirror* in October 1981. I had sent pictures of both boys' scars (with permissions from their parents) before the pressure garment treatment and at the end of the treatment to show how successful the garments had been. This was the first time I'd had anything published[65] and it was exciting.

I'd already ordered my copy of the journal from our local paper shop and rushed to collect it on the morning it arrived. But my excitement was short-lived. Two of the black-and-white pictures that I had carefully labelled "Before garment treatment" and "After garment treatment" were the wrong way round. They had labelled the nice white flat scars of Ian's arm "Ian's arm before a pressure garment has been fitted" and the raised scars "Ian, four months after the garment has been removed". I was mortified. The other pictures of

Alan were in the right order, but I had begun to realise that having something published wasn't as straightforward as it may appear.

I'd often leave the ward late in the evening when I was on a late shift, especially if I was on call for the hospital. One evening, I was called to the medical ward to see a teenager whose parents were refusing to take her home. She had a nasty weeping wound that was cancerous. She wasn't likely to live for very long and she didn't want to die in hospital.

The staff nurse took me to one side and explained the situation. "What shall I do?" she asked.

"I'll speak to the mother," I said, which I duly did, taking her to one side.

"My daughter must stay in hospital," the mother insisted.

I looked over at her daughter who was lying in her bed, holding her boyfriend's hand.

"Your daughter doesn't want to stay in hospital and we must respect her wishes," I said. "We can though make sure she has all the care that she would have in hospital at home."

I knew it was a daunting prospect for any parent but I wasn't expecting her response.

"The wound might leave stains on my new furniture. I have a new living room suite and I don't want it ruined," she said.

I was stunned, but my priority was the young girl. So I went to her and asked her what she wanted to do.

She said that she would like to go to her boyfriend's. He lived in a caravan. The boyfriend confirmed that he wanted this as well and would be quite prepared to look after her until she died. But this was *not* acceptable to the mother.

I went and telephoned the girl's consultant physician

and discussed the issue with him. He asked me if I'd hang around as he wished to come in to see the mother and he wanted me to be present.

"Of course," I said. I realised that in a situation like this, he would need the discussion witnessed.

When the consultant arrived, he discussed the girl's wishes with her. He listened to the views of the mother and of the boyfriend. He then turned to the mother.

"I've decided to discharge your daughter into the care of her boyfriend," he said.

"But she's a child," the mother protested.

"In my opinion, she's capable of making her own decision regarding her care and this is her wish, which her boyfriend fully supports. I'll arrange for a district nurse to care for her in the community."

"A caravan is *not* a suitable place for my daughter to be staying in."

"That's a risk I'm prepared to take," he responded. "The decision is between myself and my patient."

The consultant took me aside afterwards and asked for my support, should there be any comeback. I agreed, telling him that I wholeheartedly supported his decision. The girl was discharged that evening and according to the district nurse, died a few weeks later in the arms of her boyfriend.

On another winter's evening, I was again late off duty and was driving my car along the dual carriageway on my way out of Wisbech. In my headlights, I saw a man lying in the gutter, his face in a pool of blood. I stopped the car to see if I could help him. It was obvious that he was drunk.

He must've fallen and hit his nose and was now bleeding profusely. Before I could work out what to do for him, he stood up and laid himself right across the bonnet of my car.

I didn't know what to do. There was no way I could move him and there were no mobile phones in those days to call for help. I was in my sister's uniform and I tried to stop two passers-by who were walking along the pavement, but they quickly crossed over to the other side of the carriageway. I then tried to flag down passing cars, but no one would stop. It was really cold, and the man wasn't going to move because he was happy lying on my warm bonnet.

Finally, after what seemed like a long time, a police van appeared. Without speaking to me, two policemen got out of the van, removed the chap off my bonnet, threw him into the back of the van and drove away. I was quite taken aback. I took a look at the bonnet – it was blood-stained but not damaged – and drove home.

AN UNFORGETTABLE DAY

Most of the time when I was in charge of the hospital, not a lot happened. There was one day though that I will not forget. It was lunchtime on Friday, 21 September 1979. I had a phone call from the consultant responsible for the Clarkson Hospital complaining about an extremely noisy jet that had flown over Wisbech upsetting his elderly patients.

"I'd like you to telephone the RAF and make a formal complaint about this jet," he demanded. "This must *not* happen again."

A few minutes later, I was fast bleeped by the hospital switchboard and told there'd been a major incident. Two Harrier Jump Jets had collided and one of them had crashed into a housing estate in the centre of town.

One never expects to implement a major incident, though it's frequently rehearsed. I told my staff what had happened and ran to the A&E department, which had already been alerted. From there I phoned the theatres where I knew the staff would be breaking for lunch. The theatre superintendent said they'd just finished the morning lists, would cancel the afternoon list and all the staff would come to A&E to help with the casualties. I then phoned the medical unit, which I knew was less busy than the surgical one. The staff nurse on duty said they'd transfer as many patients as possible to the surgical unit to make beds available for admissions. While we were putting out the packs of notes and patient labels, casualties were beginning to arrive.

The hospital's almoner (now known as a social worker) was an enormous help. She'd grown up in Wisbech and knew everyone who came through the door, as well as who they were related to. It meant that we could put names to the numbers, which identified the casualties, and the almoner could ask about any of their relatives who may have been with them.

Many casualties arrived in shock and were given sedation to calm them down. One was the wife of the ex-mayor of Wisbech. We learnt that she was out in her garden picking a cabbage for their lunch when her house received a direct hit from the jet aircraft.

Hysterically, she was telling us, "I turned around and saw the aircraft destroy my house with my husband inside."

Another injured woman was brought in from the neighbouring house. She was in a separate room to her husband, who had come home for lunch and was with her two-year-old son, when half the house was hit. Tragically, she was the only one to survive.

In addition to the patients arriving in shock, we were receiving patients overcome with gas fumes and needing oxygen. We discovered that a gas main had been fractured.

Meanwhile, I was being bleeped constantly. I had two calls from Queen Elizabeth Hospital; one from the medical director offering to send medical staff over to help, the other from the nursing director offering to send nursing staff. In both cases I thanked them and told them that we had assistance from all our theatre staff and were coping very well. Both were very insistent though and an hour later bleeped me again saying, "Are you sure we can't help you?" We also had off-duty staff turning up to the hospital, and others phoning to offer help.

The support was encouraging. The problem was that offers of help were jamming the switchboard and blocking people who were enquiring about their relatives. I asked the telephone operators to thank off-duty members of staff volunteering to help and explain that we did have enough staff and were managing to cope.

Our next casualty was the pilot who had ejected from his plane and landed in Wisbech town. The ambulance service brought him to A&E as he'd injured his leg. I remember a surgeon cutting the trousers of the pilot to view his wound and asking what had happened. I thought at the time that it would not have been a question I would ask. The pilot was very polite, saying he was unable to tell him anything, addressing the surgeon as "sir". When the pilot was ready to be transferred to the ward, I suddenly had a thought and rushed ahead of him. I took the staff nurse aside, saying that one of the pilots was on his way to the ward. We quickly showed him into a side ward away from the other casualties.

It wasn't long after the pilot had been admitted to the ward that there was the sound of an aircraft in the hospital drive and an RAF helicopter landed. Two RAF medical staff rushed in, carrying a stretcher. I presumed they came from the RAF Hospital in Ely, which was near my home. The doctors asked me to take them to their pilot and I took them to the medical ward and into his cubicle. They quickly lifted the pilot from the bed on to their stretcher and ran from the hospital. As the helicopter lifted into the air, I could see a line of ambulances waiting. The helicopter had completely blocked the hospital entrance.

I remember two other casualties well. One was a lady who came in by ambulance in a fur coat. She was not happy to part with it on arrival in A&E. Then we discovered that she was wearing nothing underneath. Apparently, when part of her house collapsed she was in the bath. Desperate not to be seen in the nude, she managed to crawl through to her spare room and grab a coat from the wardrobe to cover herself before the emergency staff arrived to retrieve her from the rubble. The nursing staff found her a theatre gown and some paper pants so that she could be examined modestly.

The other casualties I remember well were a mother and her baby. We were told that the baby had been in her cot for an afternoon nap when part of their house was destroyed. The mother was brought to A&E extremely distressed, clutching her baby to her. Later reports of the incident told us what had happened. The BBC interviewed a neighbour who was hanging out her washing.

"There was a great shudder – then there was silence. I heard a woman's voice saying over and over again, 'My baby's dead, my baby's dead,'" she said.[66]

The baby's cot sides had protected her from injury, though she looked very dishevelled and was covered in dust. She was admitted to Jubilee Ward and examined thoroughly by our paediatrician. She stayed overnight with her mother for regular observations but was able to be discharged the following morning, having sustained nothing more than cuts and bruises. I shared this poor mother's relief that her baby was unharmed.

BBC News that night told us more about the incident. We hadn't had time to piece the events together, even though we'd been right in the thick of it. The report said that an RAF plane had crashed into two houses in a Cambridgeshire town, killing two men and a two-and-a-half-year-old boy. Two Harrier jump jets – both from the nearby air base at Wittering – collided at about 8,000 feet during a training exercise. Both pilots ejected safely. One plane broke up in mid-air and landed harmlessly in a field but the other dropped into the centre of Wisbech, destroying two houses and a bungalow. Several people were injured in the accident, including a mother and her baby who were in one of the semi-detached houses hit by the jet. The Harrier that hit the town left a crater where it landed. The crater was 15 feet wide by 50 feet deep. The Harrier narrowly missed two schools and the town's college of further education in adjoining streets.

The *Wisbech Standard* had a photo of the huge crater and the rescue workers who formed a human chain to remove bricks and rubble looking for people who were trapped. It apparently took them eight hours to recover the bodies. RAF workers dug throughout the night trying to recover some of the Harrier wreckage. I learnt too more about the mother and baby I had been caring for. The newspaper reported one of the most heroic acts. It occurred when a lady "risked her own life to save an 18-month-old baby girl dragging her to safety before part of 5, Ranmoth Road came crashing down".[67]

What I remember most about this whole major incident is how calm and organised the staff were. There was never any panic. Everyone worked together and committed themselves to the task in hand. They were amazing.

On 19 December 1979, Staff Nurse Duffy and her colleagues arranged the ward's usual annual Christmas party. They had lots of connections with firms in Wisbech and supportive people who would fund the event. This year, the crazy clown was to be the entertainer and Staff Nurse Duffy insisted that I brought my children to the party, which I did. They enjoyed it very much and saw for the first time where their mum worked.

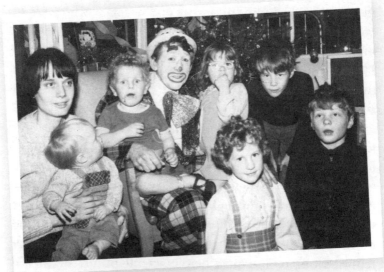

Jubilee Ward Christmas Party with the crazy clown and my three children on the right.

(Photo taken by John Day and reprinted with permission – John Elworthy, Editor, *Wisbech Standard*)

Discussions had been going on for a while about closing both the A&E department and the children's ward at North Cambridgeshire Hospital and moving the two services to Queen Elizabeth Hospital in King's Lynn. Although Wisbech had a large population, about three-quarters the size of King's Lynn, the latter had a new purpose-built hospital and was only 15 miles from the centre of Wisbech. Local people were very unhappy about these closures as they appreciated both services. Clement Freud, the local Liberal MP, raised the local people's concerns in Parliament, but the decision wasn't reversed.

Jubilee Ward was to close on 14 April 1980. The management in King's Lynn were in talks with staff over their redeployment. Staff Nurse Duffy was looking forward to retiring. I was concerned about my future. The children's ward at King's Lynn Hospital already had a ward sister who had been in post for many years and it was felt inappropriate to redeploy me to that ward. I was offered relief work for six months. There was a shortage of sisters in some areas and relief work would be a good way of introducing me to the hospital and eventually finding me a suitable ward to manage.

As this would be a new role in a different hospital, I was asked to supply two references. Miss Bradder was happy to give me one, and Miss Muirhead wrote to say that she was sorry I was being redeployed due to government cuts but would be very pleased to give me a reference. She added that it was such a pity Littleport was so far from London as they had a vacancy on Rose Gallery. They'd just opened a 12-bedded paediatric intensive care unit and their volume of work was increasing significantly. (I was thrilled for the hospital that their facilities had improved.) She hoped very much that I'd find a position I enjoyed.

Staff Nurse Duffy and her team were making plans for a closing party for Jubilee Ward. So many local people offered help or funding, including the Wisbech football supporters, the local schools, the amateur dramatic society, the local police and the local Liberal Party, as well as local shops and individuals. It was quite amazing. Eighty-four children attended the party. The principle guest was Anglia Television announcer, Christine Webber.

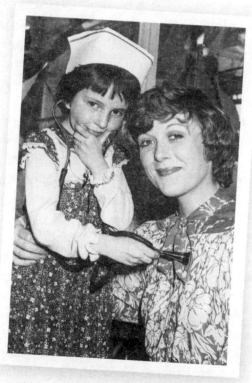

Christine Webber at the Jubilee Ward closing party.

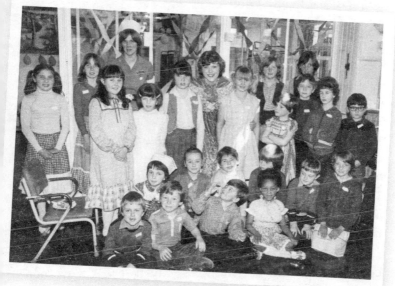

Jubilee Ward closing party.

There was a mix of entertainment – from a magician to two local singers accompanying themselves on guitars to the Wisbech Operatic and Dramatic Society. Food was in abundance and gifts were given to every child. Plaques and scrapbooks had been made for the medical and nursing staff and were presented at the end of the party. It was an unforgettable occasion, but I wasn't involved in the organisation. Staff Nurse Duffy was, as usual, very considerate of me and felt I had enough to do. It was a sad occasion for the local people who would quite obviously miss the local children's service.

Yet again I was moving on. This time it was to the newly built Queen Elizabeth Hospital, King's Lynn, near Sandringham, where the Queen spends her winter holiday.

QUEEN ELIZABETH
HOSPITAL, KING'S LYNN

I packed up my Jubilee Ward office at Wisbech on 14 April 1980 and made the journey over to King's Lynn on the same day. I was now working full-time and was to take temporary charge of two different areas for the first three months to cover for sickness and holidays. My first was a women's medical ward, where I worked for one month. The second was the adult dressings unit that I oversaw for two months. Any surgical ward could discharge patients after 24 hours and book them in to have dressings here as an outpatient. The unit was also used for patients requiring an endoscopy (examination of the inside of part of their body) or a biopsy (the removal of a piece of tissue for examination). There was a reception and a waiting area and numerous cubicles where these procedures took place. It was well-staffed and an interesting area in which to work. I had to oversee the running of the area but was also able to perform dressings and assist with the endoscopies and biopsies.

For the last three months of my relief work, I was asked if I would take charge of the male urology ward. Their ward sister had just left so I realised that they might be looking for a replacement. This ward reminded me of my time on the male urology ward at Hammersmith Hospital. I made sure that patients confined to bed had their bottles emptied more frequently, as I remembered how cheeky the men were at overfilling them at the Hammersmith.

What was different about this ward was that the urology consultant was very strict. He'd been an army surgeon during the Second World War and was trained in discipline. The junior staff on his team came in and studied the patients' notes before the ward round so they could answer all his questions, They also collected all the laboratory results well in advance of him coming.

I remember very well one incident that occurred on this ward. One evening, following a busy surgical list, a staff nurse came to me and told me that a patient was bleeding badly. We tried to stop the bleeding in every way we knew how. Eventually, I called the senior house officer, who was the first on call and the most junior doctor on the team. He was unsure about what to do next so I suggested he called the registrar, who came promptly.

The registrar examined the patient and agreed that we'd done everything we could to try to stop the bleeding. They were pondering. I knew the next step was to call the consultant who had done the operation. The registrar looked nervous.

"I really think you should call the consultant," I said to him. "If not, I will."

No one moved so I picked up the phone and asked switchboard to contact Mr T. When he answered his phone, I told him about his patient and that he was needed urgently as we couldn't stop him bleeding. I said that we and his team had tried everything we could.

I knew he was strict, but I hadn't realised just how rude he was. He began shouting at me. His language was so loud and so indecent that I held the telephone away from my ear. When he stopped shouting, I responded as calmly as I could.

"I am about to go off duty, Mr T," I said. "This patient is now *your* responsibility."

And with that, I put the phone down.

The registrar asked me if I thought the consultant was going to come to the hospital.

"He *has* to come!" I said and I went home.

It was midnight and John and I were in bed asleep. The phone rang and John answered it as he thought it might be for him. The urology consultant was on the phone and asked to speak to me. John handed me the phone with a puzzled look on his face.

"I just thought you'd like to know, Sister Martin, that I took your patient back to theatre and found he was bleeding from a major vessel. I have now managed to repair the vessel. If I hadn't, this man would have died." He then rang off.

Nothing was said to me at work the next day and the next few weeks passed as if nothing had happened. Then one day Mr T took me aside.

"Sister Martin," he said. "Would you ever consider applying for the job as my ward sister?"

Without a second's thought, I replied, "No, I would not. I don't think I could work with you, Mr T."

It wasn't long before another opportunity arose. I was told by hospital managers that there was a vacancy for a ward sister on the ophthalmic (eye) and ENT ward. My immediate reaction was to tell them that although I had

ENT experience, I'd practically no experience working with patients with eye complaints. They replied that they would like me to meet the ward consultants, which I agreed to do. I got on well with all of them and they appeared to want me to apply for this post. The two ophthalmic consultants both assured me that they would teach and support me on the ward. I applied and was accepted for the post.

All the wards in the hospital were named after local villages. This ward was called Pentney Ward and was a 28-bedded mixed sex ward with four bays and four cubicles. There were in fact three specialities of patients on the ward, as we had a maxillofacial consultant who specialised in facial problems. He was commonly referred to as the "maxfax consultant".

The eye consultants insisted that their patients were to be nursed separately from the ENT and maxfax patients to prevent cross infection. The eye patients were nursed in the bay nearest to the nurses' station. Along the corridor leading to the ward was an ophthalmic examination room. Here, not only were our own patients examined but emergencies were sent to us from A&E to be examined and either treated or admitted to the ward.

We were fully staffed as a ward, which I appreciated. I had three staff senior nurses at today's equivalent of a band 6, as well as junior staff nurses at band 5 and state enrolled trained nurses. We had students on regular placements mentored by the staff nurses and visited regularly by a nurse tutor allocated to the ward. This doesn't happen today.

I managed my off duty so that I worked at the busiest times, such as operating days, though I occasionally worked a night duty at a weekend to get to know the night staff and their working routine. My role was still a supervisory one, which meant I wasn't counted in the numbers for staffing, though I did help out with nursing duties whenever I could.

The Salmon nursing management structure had been implemented at Queen Elizabeth Hospital. There was a senior nursing officer in our section with a number of nursing officers working under her. Each nursing officer was responsible for five wards, and our nursing officer visited us on occasions, just to check we were alright. I never ever saw the senior nursing officer, who was responsible for acute services, come to the wards in the nine and a half years I worked at King's Lynn. This was unfamiliar to me as I was used to working under a knowledgeable and very visible matron who covered the whole of the hospital.

The ward had theatre lists morning and afternoon on weekdays and a high turnover of routine patients. Broken noses and broken jaws from fights kept the ENT and maxillofacial surgeons busy during some weekends. Road traffic accidents kept the ophthalmic surgeons busy until the introduction of seat belts, when numbers were reduced markedly. The one thing that we did *not* like were the bungy cords that held luggage in place on the roof racks of cars. They could come loose at one end and cause very nasty eye injuries. The eye surgeons wanted them banned.

Our routine surgical admissions were either admitted the night before for a morning list, or on the morning for an afternoon list. I would regularly do a "round" of all the ward patients and check that they knew what was happening to them that day or what to expect the next day. I would answer any questions they had. I would also tell them which registered nurse was responsible for them during that shift, but that I was always available if there was a problem. I remember sitting with one patient who was waiting for an ENT operation and asking her if she'd had an operation before. I was telling her how we would prepare her and what would happen to her. I noticed two of my staff in the background jumping up and down, trying to attract my attention.

I went to speak to them.

"Do you realise that this lady is a GP?" one of them asked.

"No," I said. "Thank you for telling me."

I went back to the patient. "I do apologise," I said. "I had no idea you were a GP. I'm sorry I've told you things you must already know."

"Please don't apologise, Sister," she said graciously. "I've never had an operation before. I actually had no idea what to expect and I really appreciated what you were telling me. Please don't stop giving these explanations to patients just because they're healthcare professionals."

Although there weren't many official doctors' rounds, it was very important in my supervisory role that I was available every time the consultants or registrars appeared on the ward. The member of trained staff allocated to care for that patient might be in theatre or with another patient and be unable to be present. The medical staff might be telling a patient that they'd done something different in the way of surgery, or even be making decisions about another form of treatment, as well as deciding when a patient should be discharged. It was so important that a senior member of staff noted what was said to patients. Unless the allocated nurses were around to accompany me with the doctors, I would then liaise with them and we'd make sure that all decisions were acted on and that the patient understood fully what had been said.

Having five consultants, all with lists at different times, kept me on my toes. There was one consultant who hated having to wait for a patient to arrive in theatre, so I was often taking them down myself to save any trouble or acrimony. He changed his tune when he became a patient himself. He finally realised that we relied on a porter with a trolley getting to us so that we could get the patient to theatre. Once again, it was clear that it really is different to be on the receiving end.

What I found strange on this adult ward was that the patients, who were admitted at 8 a.m. for the 2 p.m. operating list, were asked to take off their clothes and put them in the locker by the bed. They were then dressed in a hospital gown, open at the back, and asked to get into bed. There they would stay waiting in their bed to be examined by the senior house officer until they were called to go to theatre.

My children's training was influencing me. No child on my children's wards was ever given a gown to wear until their premedication was due. They would never have coped with sitting around in gowns. All the children were up and dressed every day. I discussed this with the staff. They too could see no good reason why the patients should be put in a gown and confined to bed for all that time.

I then discussed it with the senior house officers. They were quite adamant that patients shouldn't be allowed to remain in their clothes. They also felt that, if patients were waiting in their beds, they could rush in and examine them at a time suited to them. I tried to make them see it from the patient's point of view.

"Would you like to be sitting in a bed for up to five hours in an open-backed gown, waiting to be examined?" I asked. "We should respect our patients and allow them to keep on their own clothes," I added. "The consultants are operating on their faces. If you want to listen with a stethoscope to their chests, they can lift a shirt or a blouse for you to do that."

Eventually the senior house officers all agreed to give it a try and to their credit, none of them ever complained. It became routine to see most of our patients up and dressed. Later, I even persuaded the consultants to allow the patients to sit with a relative in the reception area downstairs until we called them for their admission examination. Patients were definitely less anxious going to theatre. I also encouraged them to be up and dressed the morning after their operation if they were well enough. They appeared to recover more quickly.

My own staff teased me as I would make sure the elderly ophthalmic patients were out of bed and dressed each morning. I even put their shoes on for them so that they could walk more comfortably to the toilet. The staff reckoned that I saw them all as children. I received many comments from other wards about this practice. Their ward sisters asked me how I was able to allow all my patients to be up and dressed. Pentney was becoming a ward that didn't conform to the practices of the other wards.

Meanwhile, I was trying to improve my knowledge about the medical conditions on the ward. I first contacted the

Ophthalmic Nurses Association and their president was incredibly helpful. She told me to contact them if there was any way that they could help me and began sending me their monthly newsletters. They even made me an honorary member of their association and invited me to their conferences.

I discovered that I couldn't do any ophthalmic training without enrolling at Moorfields Eye Hospital in London, where they offered a postgraduate course that would take at least a year. However, I did find that Queen Elizabeth Hospital in Birmingham did a distance learning diploma in ENT nursing. I would only need to travel to Birmingham to take the examination. I enrolled for the "Midland Institute" diploma course and bought the reading material. I did the distance learning by post in my own time. The course also involved my having to observe some of the ENT operations in theatre, which my consultant surgeons were very happy for me to do. I was even encouraged to scrub for one of the operations. When it came to the examination, I even enjoyed the viva (when a consultant fires questions at you) that had unsettled me so much at the end of my obstetrics course at Hammersmith Hospital. I found I could answer the questions quite easily.

Throughout this course, my staff nurses had been incredibly supportive. We had discussed the practicalities of them taking the course themselves. I knew that they would have no problems academically, but didn't wish to leave out the state enrolled nurses (SENs). I asked Queen Elizabeth Hospital in Birmingham if SEN-trained nurses could enrol on this course and was told that they could.

I discussed this with our nurse tutor, who liaised with

the nursing school, and they were encouraging. They told me that to make this course official, I should be tutoring my staff within the School of Nursing and on the ward under their direction. To do this, they wanted me to do the nine-month English National Board Teaching and Assessing Course so that I had a qualification that would make me eligible to formally teach. It would also allow me to examine our students in their practical assessments for their final exams.

It was nine months before I could officially begin teaching ENT, though informally we were teaching all the time. For almost three years I was then the co-ordinator and lecturer for the ENT course. Twelve of my staff completed the course and eight of them took and passed the examination. We became the experts used by the nursing school to teach tracheostomy care to staff in other areas of the hospital. One day, I was asked by our nursing school if I would teach ENT to student nurses at Addenbrooke's Hospital in Cambridge. I was given a small honorarium by Addenbrooke's and released by my hospital for one day a week for five months to do this. Following this, they took the overheads I used for teaching to use themselves.

A private hospital had been built in the grounds of our hospital within near walking distance. One day, a patient collapsed in this hospital and needed an emergency tracheostomy. Our on-call ENT consultant was fast bleeped and asked to give advice. He insisted that this patient was brought to our ward by blue light ambulance. We were now beginning to be so trusted by our consultants that they would not have their ENT patients nursed anywhere else.

The good thing about having nursing staff with the ENT diploma was that they were also trusted by the consultants to do procedures that were normally done by their junior doctors. We had quite a few patients admitted from A&E with an epistaxis (a serious nosebleed). It was routine that these patients would have their nostrils packed with gauze soaked in medicine to constrict the nasal vessels. My senior staff and I became so proficient at performing this procedure that these patients were sent directly to the ward rather than being kept in A&E.

I was continuing to learn about ophthalmic conditions. Along with all my trained staff, I was confident in dealing with eyes, even down to taking out a false eye, cleaning and returning it to its socket. Our ophthalmic registrar, Miss Hebbar, was excellent at her job and very keen to teach us all. When we weren't too busy, she involved us in her discussions and the treatment of patients, particularly those who came to us from A&E. In our examination room, I was taught how to use the slit lamp – a microscope with a bright light that enabled us to examine eyes in detail. It was fascinating to be able to see the incredible structure of the iris, the coloured part of the eye.

Patients regularly attended the ward needing injections into their eye, which was the most successful way of giving some treatments. On one occasion, we had three patients needing regular subconjunctival injections (into the thin tissue covering the eye) with which I was assisting. The senior house officer giving these injections was always in a hurry. After I had given the drops to numb their eyeball, he was impatient to give the injection and often gave it too quickly. The patients obviously did *not* like this.

One morning a patient asked: "Why can't you give the injections, Sister? You'd be far gentler."

I discussed this with Miss Hebbar, who was eager to teach me. She took time out to oversee me performing the procedure. I then began to do these injections on a regular basis.

One nightshift, Miss Hebbar was the registrar on call. She told me that her senior house officer was off sick and she was worried about being in the hospital all night as she had a busy clinic in the morning. She asked me if I'd look after any casualties for her that were transferred from A&E to our examination room.

"If for any reason you need my help," she said, "I'll come back to the hospital immediately."

There was only one patient that night. He had grit in his eye, and this was causing him great pain. I could see in the slit lamp that the grit had caused a cut across the cornea in the front of his eye. This was something we saw frequently. By lifting his eyelid over a two pence piece, I had a good view of the underside of the lid. I could see the offending piece of grit and removed it. I irrigated (washed out) his eye and double padded it so that he would be unable to blink. I then gave him an appointment to see Miss Hebbar so that she could assess his eye again. On his return, we were both pleased that the wound had completely healed.

My staff were very sociable and loved partying. They would really enjoy Christmas and national celebrations, decorating the ward as well as their uniform hats. If anyone had a birthday, all the staff would have a whip round for a present and a party and everyone would be invited, doctors and cleaners included.

Our ward cleaner was very much part of our team. She took such a pride in its cleanliness and the ward was always spotless. Bathrooms and toilets were cleaned morning and afternoon, the ward was damp-dusted daily, and the curtains around the beds and at the windows were changed and sent regularly to the laundry. We weren't allowed to touch anything we spilt on the floor; she was there with her mop to sort it out, however nasty it was.

It was a sad day when all the cleaning in hospitals was privatised. The firm that took over the cleaning did a ward clean once a week. Our's was done on a Friday when we had the fewest patients going to theatre. The firm would come in with electric floor cleaners, move all the beds while the other cleaning staff damp-dusted and cleaned toilets and bathrooms. If you needed any other cleaning done at any time you had to contact the service manager. I remember having a patient who'd had an infection being discharged from a cubicle. I had a patient waiting to be admitted to that cubicle and I waited for four hours for it to be cleaned. Normally, the walls and windows would be washed as well as the floor and the curtains removed for cleaning. I had to insist that these cleaners did all those jobs. The ward was never the same again.

We had many patients with cancer who required surgery. One of the major operations was the removal of the larynx (voice box). It was called a laryngectomy. These were long operations that took up a whole ENT operating list. During one of these lists, our ENT senior house officer was fast bleeped to go to the casualty department. A child had collapsed with a suspected blockage in his throat. By the time the senior house officer arrived in A&E, the child had gone into respiratory arrest and was blue. Without a second thought, the senior house officer took the child in his arms and ran with him up the stairs and into the theatre where our senior ENT consultant was performing one of these major operations. He apparently just placed the child on top of the adult patient on which the consultant was operating, and the consultant performed an emergency tracheostomy on the child, saving his life.

The child was examined properly after the theatre list had been completed and found to have an abscess located at the back of his throat. This was life-threatening. I'd experienced a child with one of these abscesses when I was a first-year student at GOS, working on the ENT ward. This abscess was drained on an emergency theatre list and the child given regular intravenous antibiotics. Once the course of antibiotics was finished and his tracheostomy removed, he was discharged home with no ill effects. I don't think that particular adult patient ever knew that his surgical team saved a child's life during his operation.

Laryngectomies involved the patient having to have a tracheostomy and, as their voice box had been removed, having to learn a different way of speaking through a form of burping. It was tough on the patients as it could be difficult to master, but we had a system of introducing them to a patient who'd been through the operation and learnt to talk. This past patient, who'd volunteered to give this service, was a huge support to them and visited them daily until they were discharged home.

One patient who'd had this operation was really doing well. He was determined to learn to talk and was becoming quite good at it. One evening after his wife had just left from visiting him, he said to my auxiliary nurse that he was tired and wanted an early night. He told her that he was going to have a wash down and go to bed, so he didn't need his evening drink. She came and told me what the gentleman had told her and that she would look in on him later.

Half an hour later, she pulled his emergency bell. I rushed in and saw that he'd had a cardiac arrest. I shouted for the crash trolley and started external cardiac massage while my auxiliary phoned for the crash team. They responded in record time. He was intubated and given medicines directly into his heart to try to bring him round. After 20 minutes, the crash team gave up. We then found a note on his bedside table saying how sorry he was to have done this, but he didn't want to be a burden to his family. We were all devastated that this had happened.

My phone call to his wife was one of the hardest I've ever made. She lived very near the hospital and came quickly to the ward. I couldn't help shedding some tears as I showed her his note.

Her response to me was: "Sister Martin, if *I* didn't know that this was going to happen, how on earth could *you* have known?"

We both hugged each other. It was a sad time for the ward; we all felt bereaved. It was made even worse by one member of staff bringing in the local paper, whose head-lines read "Hospital Death: Nurses Cleared". There was never any question of the staff being blamed. I had to attend the coroner's court at a later date. Even then I was only asked for the sequence of events before the gentleman's suicide note was read out.

I had a distant relationship with management. They didn't seem to know what happened on the wards. I never saw the senior nursing officer unless she called me to her office. The nursing officer for our unit came to us occasionally. She carried the crash team bleep but, when she arrived at the scene of a cardiac arrest, she never appeared to know what to do.

One day, when she came to a cardiac arrest on our ward, I felt embarrassed for her as she just stood in the background. I gave her a pen and paper and asked her to record the medicines and doses that the team were giving to the patient, which she did. Whenever I saw her at another call out, she produced a pen and paper from her pocket to record the medicines given. At least she was doing something.

One morning as I arrived on the ward, my staff nurse, who'd been on night duty, rushed up to me. She'd just given a patient a prescribed eye drop so that his eye could be examined half an hour later when she realised that he had glaucoma, a condition in which these drops should not be given. I said to her that I would ring the senior house officer, who had prescribed the drop, take a verbal order for drops to reverse the effect and we would give it to him. I knew the senior house officer would sign the prescription when he came to the ward. We gave the gentleman the second drop, telling him what had happened.

When we turned around, we found that our nursing officer had been watching us. We didn't know how long she'd been there.

"I want you to come immediately to my office," she said to my staff nurse.

As they were leaving the ward, I approached the nursing officer. "What's all this about?" I asked her.

She turned and said: "This girl has made a drug error and must be disciplined."

"It was *not* my staff nurse who made a drug error," I corrected her. "She gave exactly what was on the prescription. It was *she* who put it right. If anyone needs disciplining, it's the doctor who wrote the prescription, not her."

The nursing officer left the ward on her own, with no comment.

I was also nearly disciplined myself by the senior nursing officer. She called me to her office one morning and said that a senior charge nurse (we called male sisters charge nurses), whom I'd met for the first time the morning before, had complained about my not respecting his decision to put an emergency ENT patient with a bad nose bleed into the ophthalmic bay where she could be observed. I explained about us never mixing ENT patients with ophthalmic ones because of the risk of cross infection, which could result in an ophthalmic patient losing their sight. I asked if he had discussed this with my staff before doing so. She was not impressed with my response, so I invited her to discuss it with our senior ophthalmic surgeon. She wasn't going to do that, so I was told to leave.

The staff on the ward were always coming up with ideas as to how we could make our patients' stays a better experience. We'd put together a library of talking books for the ophthalmic patients to listen to, which they loved. I'd written quite a few patient leaflets to explain different conditions, some of which had been illustrated by a friend of mine. We had quite a collection of these patient leaflets. Some were given out to patients in the outpatient's department explaining the condition for which they needed treatment. Others were given to patients on discharge to help them look after themselves at home.

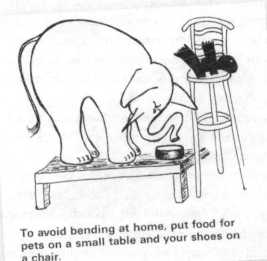

To avoid bending at home, put food for pets on a small table and your shoes on a chair.

An instruction leaflet for patients following a cataract operation.

In 1988, I decided to send a leaflet on glue ear in for a competition, as I'd had good patient feedback. It won third prize and was published in a journal called *Professional*

Nurse. It was the second time I'd had something published. This though was not where it ended. I was asked my permission for the leaflet to be reprinted in a book called *Patient Education Plus* and in another book *Child Care, Some Nursing Perspectives*. It amazed me how just coming third in a competition had led to three publications.

It was Easter 1986 and Jonathan was 18. The Sybil Elgar School told us that he had to move to an adult training centre and recommended one in Spilsby in Lincolnshire. It was about an hour and a half from us. They assured us that it had a good reputation as they'd sent youngsters there before and, because Jonathan would be a boarder, they would send a member of their staff to stay with him for a few days to ensure a good transition. We visited the centre ourselves, which was in the countryside, and were confident that the principal of the Sybil Elgar School had done her best for our son. Cambridgeshire County Council were to sponsor him, and a young, enthusiastic social worker made the arrangements.

I packed all of Jonathan's favourite things to help him feel at home as he was now going to be a full boarder. He had his new Walkman with CDs, his radio, his tape recorder with all his favourite music tapes, and his favourite books to read, as well as pictures of his family. John even gave him one of a set of hairbrushes that had belonged to his father. He was asked to bring a suit to wear on formal occasions, which we bought for him. He chose some of his special clothes to take, particularly a bright red silky shirt that he liked.

When we took Jonathan for his first term, I unpacked

his case in which I had left a list of all the clothes and items he'd taken with him. We heard nothing from the centre for a while, then halfway through the term, we were phoned by one of the staff, who said that Jonathan had run off and they couldn't find him. I said that we would come over at once, but they insisted that we shouldn't. They said they'd keep in touch with us. They phoned us a few hours later to say that they'd found him and that he was safe and well and not to worry.

Near the end of term, I answered the phone to a gentleman who said he was a psychiatrist.

"I have a request from the carers of the training centre for a prescription of haloperidol for Jonathan," he said.

I was very familiar with the effects haloperidol had on children, from using it at GOS. It was commonly known as a "chemical cosh".

"I am happy to prescribe this drug for your son," he went on. "But I want your permission to do so."

I was taken aback. The centre hadn't informed us that they were having problems with Jonathan. "When you examined Jonathan, what were his symptoms that warranted the prescribing of haloperidol?" I asked.

The gentleman said, "I haven't seen him, but I have his reports."

"When you do assess him, I'd like to be present," I said.

"I don't intend to see him," he said.

"Really?"

"I trust the carers' assessment."

"In that case," I said, "I do *not* give my permission for you to prescribe this drug to my son."

273

A few days later the psychiatrist managed to get John on the phone. He asked him if he would give his permission for the medicine to be prescribed.

John said: "If my wife won't give her permission for you to prescribe haloperidol to my son, I certainly won't."

A few weeks later we collected Jonathan for his summer holiday. Meanwhile, I'd been talking to one of our psychiatrists at the hospital whom I knew well. I told him about our phone calls and asked for his opinion. He said that generally haloperidol shouldn't be given to autistic youngsters but asked me how would I feel if he prescribed the smallest of doses for us to try during our summer holiday to see what effect it had on him. John and I agreed.

We tried this very small dose on Jonathan while we were all having a family boating holiday. He was completely zombified, interspersed with an unusual number of fierce tantrums and was clearly in distress. I stopped the medicine, but it took around three weeks before it ceased to affect Jonathan. I reported back to our psychiatrist when I returned to work. He said I was right to refuse permission for the Spilsby psychiatrist to prescribe the medicine for Jonathan, as it clearly was *not* suitable for him.

After the holiday, Jonathan was due to return to Spilsby. We were both anxious about him. John was to take him as I was on duty. As John was about to leave Jonathan, he asked him repeatedly if he was sure he wanted to stay, but Jonathan said "Yes" each time. Feeling uneasy, John left him but then caught sight of him coming out of the building. He watched him lean against a wall with his head in his hand.

"I don't know if I did the right thing leaving him there," John said to me on his return.

When I came back from work, I got a phone call from the centre. Jonathan had run off again and the police had been informed.

This time I phoned the local Lincolnshire police. "I gather you've had a call to say that my son, Jonathan Martin, has run away from the adult training centre in Spilsby?"

"We're having difficulty finding him, Mrs Martin," the officer said. "Can you give us a description of Jonathan? What was he wearing?"

"He's fair-haired and he's wearing a light blue T-shirt and navy blue trousers. His dad and I are planning to drive over as we're concerned about him."

There was a pause. Then the policeman said, "I don't think that will be necessary."

"Why?" I asked.

"The centre gave us a completely different description. They even told us he had dark hair. We've had a report of a lad that does match the description of your son and we're sending a panda car to collect him now." He added: "We'll contact you as soon as we've picked him up."

About a fortnight after this incident, we were summoned by the centre and told that they wanted to meet with us. We drove over on a day when we were both free. On arrival, we were ushered into a room where a number of people were already seated round an oval polished table. Jonathan was dressed in his posh suit and his nice social worker was present. The principal told us about some of the things that Jonathan had been doing while he was at the centre. Among them was taking himself up into their attic and hiding. But a far more disturbing tale was how he'd tried to throw himself in front of a moving car.

"Why weren't we told all this at the time?" John asked.

"He's never behaved like this before," I added.

"Mr and Mrs Martin," the principal began, "we don't feel that the centre is the right place for Jonathan, but we're happy to keep him here until a more suitable placement can be found."

John and I, who were not sitting together, stood up simultaneously. We both said together: "We'll take him now!"

I went with Jonathan's social worker and a carer to his room to collect his belongings. I took his case from the top of the wardrobe and got out the list of his belongings. I looked round the room and opened drawers and the wardrobe. All I could find was a few underclothes, a couple of pairs of trousers and a shirt or two. I was shocked.

"Where are the rest of his clothes?" I asked the carer. "Where's his Walkman, his radio, his tape recorder, all his tapes and CDs and the hairbrush his dad gave him? Even the pictures of his family have gone. I want these things found now!"

Jonathan's social worker was as shocked as I was.

The carer went away to find someone. When she returned, she said: "We don't understand where his belongings have gone."

"These articles must be found and returned to Jonathan's family," the social worker told her, quite firmly on our behalf.

He turned to me. "I *will* try to make sure Jonathan's belongings are returned to him."

When we were outside, I spoke to the social worker: "It looks to me as though Jonathan has been bullied. *All* his belongings that were *so* important to him and helped him to feel secure … they've been systematically taken from him. How can this have happened *without them knowing?*"

"I agree," he said. "I'm going back now to report this to Cambridgeshire County Council. It mustn't be allowed to happen to anyone else." He then promised he'd do his utmost to find a secure placement for our son.

We took Jonathan home.

Weeks later a small parcel came in the post. It was Jonathan's favourite red shirt with all the buttons torn off it. The note inside said: "This is all that we can find of Jonathan's belongings."

The social worker was true to his word. He found Jonathan a very sought-after place in Camphill Community, Colig Elidyr in South Wales. We were very fortunate. These communities are grounded in the principles of "inclusion, mutual respect and increasing life chances of people with autism, learning difficulties and disability".[68] Although Colig Elidyr normally took youngsters from 16 to 19 after their secondary education, they agreed to take Jonathan until he was 22.

We were asked to take Jonathan to meet their clinical psychologist for an assessment before he started there. She lived on the south coast and was an advisor to the Camphill movement. As the return trip would take a whole day, we decided that John would take him so that I could fit my working shift around looking after our children.

Later, John told me how the interview went. "The psychologist was elderly," he said, "but very shrewd. She watched Jonathan for a short while and then told me how she believed he behaved. She was right. She asked if he was sensitive to medicines and I told her about the haloperidol. She was appalled that it had been suggested and told me how it would have affected Jonathan. She was right again. She said that the Spilsby psychiatrist had described Jonathan's autism as 'infantile schizophrenia', which showed that he was seriously out of date. She confirmed that Jonathan would be offered a place at the Camphill Community, and she thought it would be the right placement for him."

Jonathan started his three years at Colig Elidyr in 1987 and enjoyed his time there.

In August 1987, I learnt that the sister of Rudham Ward, the paediatric ward that was adjacent to Pentney, had been suspended. I didn't know her well as I'd had very little to do with her. I understood that she had run the ward for many years and long before the new hospital had been built. I also knew that she had an MBE for rescuing children during flooding at the old hospital. I was asked by management and the paediatric consultants if I would oversee the running of Rudham Ward as well as my own ward. I thought it would only be for a short time, so I agreed. What I noticed was how low the morale of the staff was, which I put down to the suspension of their sister.

As Christmas approached, the staff nurses came to see me on Pentney Ward. I remember one of them saying: "How come your ward is so beautifully decorated? Where did you get all these lovely decorations?" I told her that the Friends of the Hospital gave each ward £25 a year for decorations and we'd been accumulating them over the years. That was why we had so many.

It wasn't until the middle of 1988, a year later, that I was told that a new sister was needed for the ward. The paediatricians began to ask me if I would consider leaving Pentney Ward and coming to work full-time on Rudham. I now knew them well from working as their temporary ward sister. They also knew that I was Great Ormond Street-trained. I was very happy on Pentney and had built up a really good team of staff. I would be very sad to leave it but I decided eventually that perhaps a new challenge would be good for me and that it would be an opportunity to work in my beloved paediatrics again. I said I would apply for the post and was accepted.

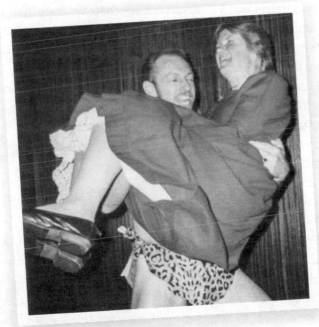

My leaving party from Pentney Ward.

Leaving Pentney Ward was hard for me. I'd been working on the ward for eight years. The staff appeared not to want me to go. They convinced me to have a leaving party and we arranged it in a local restaurant. We had a good turnout of nursing and medical staff with their partners.

The restaurant was decorated with balloons and bunting. We had a lovely meal. After that, I was presented with a gold watch, to which the medical staff had contributed generously. Then the staff began partying. It was all going well with lots of dancing and drinking when there was suddenly a silence. I worried that the staff had arranged a surprise for me. Suddenly, the partner of one of my staff appeared dressed as Tarzan, or perhaps I should say he was hardly dressed! Claiming I was his Jane, he began to lift me and throw me around the room. I was somewhat embarrassed, but they were obviously enjoying this.

I really enjoyed Pentney Ward and it's a ward I won't forget. To this day I still send Christmas cards and hear from some of the staff.

RETURN TO NURSING CHILDREN

I officially took up the post of sister on Rudham Ward in August 1988. This time, I was able to have a period of orientation back into paediatrics, arranged at Addenbrooke's in Cambridge, where I spent three weeks on their paediatric unit. I was encouraged by the formal letter of acceptance I received from our senior nursing officer for the post of ward sister. Not only was she offering me this period of reorientation, but her concluding paragraph read: "I look forward to you taking up this appointment and if there is any way I can be of any help, I hope you will not hesitate to contact me."

What had changed most in paediatric centres was the development of paediatric intensive care units (PICUs). I was to spend most of my orientation in the Addenbrooke's PICU. I'd already experienced the adult intensive care unit at Brompton Hospital. Miss Muirhead had written to me in 1980, telling me that they had just opened a new 12-bedded PICU in that hospital. These units were managed by a team led by a paediatric consultant and a paediatric consultant anaesthetist. Now I was to experience working on a unit like this and I was looking forward to it.

What I found when I began working on the unit was that the equipment was becoming even more sophisticated. Not only were there heart monitors, which we'd had in our high dependency bay on Rose Gallery, but there were also machines measuring children's blood oxygen levels and blood gases. This meant that the simple charts we'd had at the bottom of each child's bed when I trained at GOS had expanded into something much more complex. They were, though, giving a lot more vital information at a glance about the condition of seriously ill children. The ventilators too were now more compact and children were kept alive with conditions that they would not have survived previously.

It was on this unit that I met Fraser. He was born with multiple problems. His diaphragm, which should separate his chest cavity from the rest of his abdominal organs, had an opening, allowing some of the organs from his abdomen to move up into his chest cavity. As a result of this, he was born with only one lung, that lung only having half its function, so he couldn't breathe without a tracheostomy and a ventilator. Lung transplants weren't an option in those days.

All Fraser's initial surgery and care had taken place at GOS. He'd recently been transferred to Addenbrooke's PICU to be nearer his family. His home happened to be in King's Lynn and it soon became clear to me that Fraser's mum rarely visited him. This was preventing both her and Fraser bonding together. His mum was a single mother with an older child and was living on income support, so she had a huge amount on her plate on top of her sick son.

The PICU staff were keen for me to get to know Fraser and take over some of his care in the hope that he could be transferred to Rudham Ward. Doing so was really enjoyable for me. I found that in spite of all his problems, Fraser was a bright, alert child. He'd had two operations at GOS, one at 13 days old and a second when he was two months. He was now five months. He'd gone through a great deal in his short life. He was now in a position where he was likely to have to live attached to a ventilator with a tracheostomy indefinitely, if he was going to survive at all.

Throughout those few weeks at Addenbrooke's Hospital, I was pondering about what was best for Fraser. I worried about whether a ward such as Rudham – a 30-bedded general paediatric ward – was capable of coping with a child like him, yet he needed to be nearer his family. The previous ward sister on Rudham didn't have paediatric training – in fact, there had never been a paediatric nurse on the ward, just like on Jubilee Ward in Wisbech. I also learnt that during a previous practice placement audit, which the English National Board had done to assess whether the ward was a suitable place for students to do their six-week children's placement, it was suggested that students would be removed from the ward. I realised I had a lot of work to do in order to build up the competencies of the staff and the reputation of my new ward.

Rudham Ward specialised in general paediatric medicine, surgery, orthopaedics and ENT, as well as day surgery. As on Pentney, I was responsible for the ward budget, which included assessing the amount of equipment used and justifying what was ordered. On my first day, I noticed that as in Wisbech the crash trolley was only suitable for adults, not children. I realised then that the staff probably had little experience in resuscitating a child. I also noticed that the blood pressure machines only had adult cuffs, so I presumed again that blood pressure readings were rarely taken. I ordered paediatric cuffs anyway. I didn't have a Senior Staff Nurse Duffy who'd been on the ward for years, but I had state enrolled nurses who had. I tried to utilise them with our staff nurses in training our students, who luckily hadn't yet been removed from the ward when I arrived. Many of the staff nurses lacked confidence and I needed somehow to restore this.

As Christmas approached and ward decorating began, I realised how few decorations we had. I asked for staff volunteers to buy what they thought was needed with the Friends of the Hospital's £25 budget. They came back with a huge amount, all apparently bargains. Parents were also showering the staff with Christmas gifts. We were getting so many chocolates that at one of the ward staff meetings, I suggested that to preserve our waistlines, we might lock them in the store cupboard and each member of staff take one home at Christmas. We did that and the staff were thrilled to choose a box each. We even had enough left over to open and share with the medical staff on Christmas Day.

I'd always enjoyed teaching, especially in small groups, and since doing the teaching and assessing course, I'd been doing a lot more. We began to have regular formal teaching sessions on Rudham Ward. As I suspected, Addenbrooke's PICU paediatrician had been talking to our paediatricians, asking about the possibility of Fraser being transferred to our ward. His mum was still only able to visit him about once a month. Our paediatricians discussed this with me. My staff were unfamiliar with nursing children with a tracheostomy and ventilators and, as I suspected, had rarely needed to resuscitate a child. I had to start teaching these competencies. I taught tracheostomy care, suction techniques to keep the tracheostomy clear and paediatric resuscitation. The paediatricians familiarised the staff with the ventilator Fraser would be using. It was important that the staff were prepared with all these competencies before Fraser arrived. We didn't want them to feel that they couldn't cope.

When Fraser first arrived on the ward, he was frightened and withdrawn. He began vomiting his food and losing weight. He also frightened everyone as he had frequent respiratory arrests during his short periods off the ventilator. It was a new environment for him, but he soon began to settle. In addition to these nursing problems, the finance managers were complaining to me about the cost of the equipment I was ordering and the fact that I required extra registered nursing hours to special Fraser 24 hours a day. One of the administration staff commented that he should never have been operated on as a baby. "What sort of a life will he lead?" was commonly asked. Yet the decision hadn't been ours. If Fraser was born and survived today with present medical progress, he might well have had a lung transplant.

It was a tense first few months. Our ward incorporated a philosophy of family-centred care, which encouraged parents, however sick their child, to be involved in their care themselves. Fraser's mother was reluctant to be involved in his day-to-day care. She didn't want to sleep on the ward, even though her daughter could stay too. The only care she would do for him was bathing and changing his nappy, which was familiar to her. We were trying to familiarise her with the routine care of his tracheostomy. She would have just one attempt at suction and claim she was competent.

By the time Fraser was a year old, we were concerned about his obvious hostility towards other children. He would go to the extremes of hitting and biting them. He was still in a cubicle with a nurse giving him one-to-one care and only saw other children when they ventured in to see him. I felt that being isolated from the other children was holding back his development. I suggested he should be moved into the 12-bedded ward.

My staff were reluctant to support me as they felt that management would use this as an excuse to cut our staffing levels. I reassured them that I would try not to let this happen. The medical staff were also reluctant, suggesting that if Fraser picked up an infection it could prove fatal. I persevered and it was agreed that we should have a trial period. This required extra oxygen and suction points being installed in the main ward, which made me even less popular with the finance department.

Fraser was furious about the move and sat with his back to the occupants of the ward for three days. He also refused to relate to his special nurse, which was very unusual, but he gradually came around. The other children were fascinated by his machinery and the other mothers were amazingly responsive to his charm. They began to encourage his mother, who responded to their friendship, and under their influence began to visit Fraser more frequently and take over more of his care.

In the main ward, Fraser's hardest lesson to learn was to share. Sharing his toys, his bath and worst of all his nurses, was a traumatic experience. So, to gain extra attention, he began removing his tracheostomy tube. The panic that he caused certainly got staff running. This had to stop. I enlisted the help of the occupational therapy department and they came to our rescue. They set up a specially adapted bell for him to call us, which Fraser loved. He could now get attention without resorting to the extreme of stopping himself breathing.

My next concern was Fraser's speech as I'd failed to get a speaking valve for his tracheostomy tube that worked. The speech therapy department suggested he should learn Makaton signing. That meant we all had to learn it first. With another member of my staff, I spent an intensive study day learning the rudiments of signing. Then came the task of teaching Fraser and keeping the rest of the staff up to date with his signing through regular lunchtime teaching sessions. Fraser learnt signing with exceptional speed, proving that his episodes of stopping breathing hadn't affected his ability to learn. I found it extremely hard to keep ahead of him. He practised on staff, children and their parents. He was thrilled to have a way of communicating. His mother felt very self-conscious signing and was less enthusiastic until he began signing "Mummy".

Eventually, Fraser's mother learnt to take over all her son's care. He was having longer times off his ventilator until he coped with just needing it at night. He then began to have short trips home and with the help of the paediatric district nurse, his mum's coping skills improved so much that I relaxed and felt able to support his eventual discharge home. He was to have regular follow-up visits by his paediatric district nurse. I learnt that when Fraser was five, he began to attend a special school and later was able to attend his

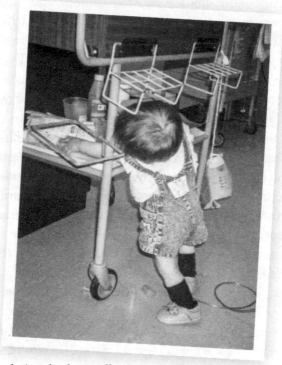

Fraser exploring the drug trolley.

local primary school. He also learnt to speak by covering his tracheostomy tube with his finger and apparently had lots of conversation![69] None of this surprised me as I always thought he was a bright little boy.

During the time that Fraser was on Rudham Ward, the skills and confidence of staff were growing. The trained staff were performing tasks that had been completely new to them. Their response to emergencies was carried out with great speed and professionalism. As their skills became acknowledged, especially by medical staff, they became more enthusiastic about teaching students and improving the reputation of the ward. The School of Nursing arranged a second placement practice audit with the English National Board and this time the ward was assessed as suitable for student placements.

Parents often benefited a lot from staying on the ward. They encouraged each other, helped the staff and, in the case of Fraser, supported Fraser's mum to be more confident with him. I remember having a problem with the parents of a seven-year-old who was on the ward for a number of weeks on traction. He made his wishes known by screaming. His parents were both protective of him and controlled by him. The staff were getting very worried by this and consistently complaining about the child.

I spoke to the parents and explained that the other children were frightened by the screams, including little Fraser. I said that if they couldn't control his screaming, my only solution would be to put their child into a side room on his own. His parents were furious, but the screaming continued. In the end I moved him to a side room and told the little boy that he could only return to the ward when he'd had a full day with no screams. After a scream-free day had passed, I returned him to the main ward. There was one time when he tried a scream, but after a threat from me to move him back into the side room he stopped. He then began to speak if he had requests or wanted attention, which actually surprised his parents as this behaviour was new to them. The staff too, who had been watching the child's reaction carefully, were also surprised at the change in the child. They'd originally been worried about the parent's fury over my moving him into a side room, but realised it had to be done.

The staff, who worked regularly in the day case ward, began to be enthusiastic about putting together a book about going to theatre for day surgery children. They felt that this would reduce the time that they spent admitting these children to the ward. The hospital photographer agreed to photograph ward areas and the theatre, and the staff they would meet, such as the doctors and the theatre porters.

Every possible way the child could be prepared and recovered from theatre was recorded and made into a book. Copies were made and these books were shared with each child and their parents on admission. As the staff had predicted, it certainly helped to reduce the time spent on admitting these children. The parents and children loved the books and as children began meeting staff, both in the ward and the operating theatre, they would point people's pictures out in the book to everyone, saying: "Is that you?"

We'd keep replying: "Yes, that is me!"

I had an interesting experience when I was on duty one Sunday. An officer in full military uniform arrived on the ward with a wheelchair full of flowers. He asked for the person in charge and told me that Her Majesty The Queen had sent these flowers for the children.

I was taken off guard. "You're joking," I said.

He stood very upright. "No, Madam, I am not," he said. "These flowers have been sent for your children by Her Majesty Queen Elizabeth."

I then realised that the Queen must have been staying at her country home in Sandringham and these flowers would've been given to her by the public when she attended church that morning. This was her equerry, the officer in attendance on the Queen. I accepted the flowers graciously and asked him to thank the Queen on behalf of the children. The children were absolutely thrilled, telling their relatives constantly during the week that they had been given a present of flowers from the Queen.

Meanwhile, there had been more change in our home life. A few years earlier, two young sisters, whose mother had died, came to live with their aunt and her husband in Littleport. When the elder girl, Jennifer, was 12, the aunt died. For more than two years, the girls continued to live with their uncle, but then social services began to look for foster parents. Our organist taught at Jennifer's school and asked us if we would consider fostering her.

After a family conference, our children agreed that we should do it. This meant that all the bedrooms in the new vicarage would be filled. When the new house was built, we'd persuaded the diocese to divide a bedroom into two, so we had two reasonable-sized rooms and three little ones. This spare bedroom would become Jennifer's, and she moved in with us.

John was involved in arranging for the younger girl, Jane, to be fostered by a couple who lived very close to the church so that there would be only a church yard between the two girls. After about six months, Jane decided that she wanted to be with her sister, lay down on the main Welney Road late one evening and screamed. We talked to Jane's foster parents and to social services.

We had another family conference. We decided, as a family, that we would also foster Jane, but they should have separate bedrooms seeing as their relationship wasn't entirely peaceful. They were quite different in personality. Jennifer was an attractive and intelligent girl, but she was secretive. My worry was that she would occasionally leave the house at about midnight. I'd follow her to make sure she was OK. I think she only wanted to be on her own for a while away from our busy household. Jane was the opposite. Lively and chatty, she told us everything. Even though she could be very fierce and feisty – as the screaming in the road episode had proved – she was straight with us.

Our house was now very full and it meant that Jonathan, being at Coleg Elidyr, would have to share a room with James when he came home for his holidays. In reality, they actually both coped very well with the arrangement. We were proud of them.

After a year or two there was to be another big change. By the end of 1989, we'd been in Littleport for 11 years. I was still enjoying the challenge of running Rudham Ward, but John was beginning to feel that he'd achieved all he could in the parishes. Our children were reaching different stages in their education: Jonathan was at Coleg Elidyr; James was taking his A-levels; and Philippa was coming up to her GCSEs. Which left Jennifer and Jane.

We had another family conference. The sisters decided they both wanted to stay in Littleport. We could understand that, so social services arranged for new foster parents who would take both girls and be near enough for them to remain at their school.

John went on to Canon Hardaker's list, who was then co-ordinating those looking to move and those looking for new clergy. The Bishop of Sheffield offered John the post of becoming team rector of Attercliffe and Darnall, a seven-year appointment. It meant not only returning to the inner city but also that John could work with a team of clergy. One of the congregations would be a combination of United Reformed Christians, Methodists and Anglicans. The Methodist or United Reform Church would take turns at appointing one of the clergy. John was looking forward to this new project.

Although I was happy to return to the inner city where the people were inclined to be very open and straight, I was sorry to leave Rudham Ward. I felt I'd made a difference there. The senior nursing officer was very quick to appoint a replacement ward sister who was paediatric trained and had just moved into the area. The new sister must have known about Rudham's past problems as she kindly reassured me that she would try to keep up Rudham's present standards, which I'm sure she did.

As I was leaving Rudham, I couldn't help but reflect on how nursing had changed my life. I'd begun the sixties as a schoolgirl, but by 1966 I had completed my children's and adult nurse training and was married. I'd been excited to be accepted for training at GOS. Gwen Kirby, our matron, was dedicated to her patients. She and the GOS ward sisters were role models who inspired us in our careers. They were respected not only for the knowledge they'd acquired in their specialist subjects, but also for the part they played in our training, caring for the health and wellbeing of their students and developing the expertise of each generation of new nurses. I was privileged to be involved in the treatment and recovery of children with rare diseases who had previously never survived. We never stopped learning.

Consultants, too, were concerned to develop our skills and share their knowledge with us. They recognised the importance of our role in children's recovery.

For those of us who were lucky enough to experience it, Hammersmith Hospital was exciting and challenging. I enjoyed living in the community with my newfound friends. On night duty we were thrown into the deep end. This was the time and place where my first experience of ward management was really tested.

The birth of my three children caused me to have a break in nursing. In 1969, my husband's work took me to Bermondsey in the East End of London. Here I was taken out of my "middle-class" comfort zone and taught to love these quick-witted people, who couldn't tolerate airs and graces, but were intensely caring to people in trouble. Eventually as my children grew, I was able to return to my beloved GOS part-time and then to Brompton Hospital as a night sister.

Another move took me to North Cambridgeshire Hospital to be in charge of my own children's ward. Here we had the Harrier disaster. I happened to be managing the hospital. People died, it was an appalling disaster and yet what impressed me was the way staff dropped everything they were doing and came together to work as a team. The response was humbling.

After the closure of our little Wisbech hospital, I spent most of the eighties working as a ward sister at Queen Elizabeth Hospital, King's Lynn. I worked with some remarkable nurses and impressive medical staff who taught me a lot. Finally I was offered the leadership of a struggling children's ward, Rudham, and the opportunity to turn it around. It was very satisfying.

The next stage of my life, in Sheffield, was to be a watershed. My first experience was to make me question whether I had a future in nursing at all, but as yet, I had no conception of the care that could be achieved as part of a multidisciplinary team, given the right management and dedicated colleagues. That book is being written even now.

REFERENCES

1. Wikipedia – Kensington Roof Gardens. Accessed October 2020 at: https://enwikipedia.org/wiki/Kensingtonroofgardens
2. Telfer, K. (2008) *The Remarkable Story of Great Ormond Street Hospital*. Simon & Schuster 14–18.
3. www.gosh.org>about us>our history. Accessed 20/02/2021.
4. UK News (March 2020) "Charles's sporting injuries and minor operations over the years", *Shropshire Star*, accessed from https://www.shropshirestar.com/news/uknews/2020/03/25
5. Fryer, J. (2020), "ATTEN-SHUN! The Military Rules that can change your life", *Daily Mail*, Saturday January 4th 2020.
6. HHARP, Historic Hospital Admissions Records Project. "The History of the Hospital for Sick Children, Great Ormond Street (1852–1914)". Accessed November 2019 from: *Historical background GOSH*.
7. Barnes, E. (2009) "Cancer coverage: the public face of childhood leukaemia in 1960s Britain". *Endeavour 2008* Mar.: 32(1); 10–15.
8. Public Health England (2019) "Tetanus in England: 2018"; *Health Protection* Report; 13; 10; 22 March 2019.
9. University of Oxford (2018) "Vaccine Knowledge Project: Tetanus", accessed May 2020 at https://vk.ovg.ox.ac.uk/vk/tetanus
10. "Advanced Paediatric Life Support – The Practical Approach (1998)", Advanced Life Support Group. BMJ Publishing Group.
11. Moncrieff, A. and Norman, A.P. (1957) *A Textbook on the Nursing and Diseases of Sick Children*, H.K. Lewis & Co. Ltd., London.
12. Graham, G. (1993) Obituary: Dr Mildred Creak, *Independent* accessed October 2020 at: https://independent.co.uk/news/people/obituary-dr-mildred-creak
13. Sickle Cell Society, accessed July 2020 from: sicklecellsociety.org/resource/sickle-cell-anaemia/
14. Stanford Children's Health, accessed July 2020 from: Stanfordchildrens.org

15. Lee, K.C., Joory, K. and Moiemen, N.S. (2014), "History of Burns: The past, present and the future", Burns and trauma; 2; 169–180.

16. Dupuytren's Classification from Dupuytren, G, Brierre de Boismont, A. J., Alm, P. (1839) "Oral lessons of clinical surgery, faites à l'Hotel-Dieu de Paris" Baillière Paris; cited in Lee, et al. (2014), "History of Burns".

17. Moncrieff, A.A., et al. (1964) "Lead Poisoning in Children", *Archives of Diseases in Childhood*; 39; 1; 1–13.

18. Icahn School of Medicine – Bone Lead Tests – K XRF. Accessed July 2020 from https://labs.icahn.mssm.edu/toddlab/bone-lead-test/

19. Wikipedia – Lead-based paint in the United Kingdom. Accessed October 2021 from https://en.wikipedia.org/wiki/Lead-based_paint_in_the_United_Kingdom

20. Ayyar, V.S. (2011) "History of Growth Hormone Therapy", *Indian Journal of Endocrinology and Metabolism*, 15 (Suppl.3); S162–S165.

21. Elborn, S. (2018) "The History, and the Future, of Cystic Fibrosis. The Early Years", Royal Brompton and Harefield NHS Foundation Trust. Accessed April 2020 at https://www.rbht.nhs.uk/blog/history-and-future-cystic-fibrosis

22. Robin, P. (1923) "La chute de la base de la langue considérée comme une nouvelle cause de gene dans la respiration naso-pharyngienne". *Bull Acad Med Paris*; 89; 37–41. Cited in Wagener, et al. 2002.

23. Robin, P. (1934) "Glossoptosis due to atresia and hypertrophy of the mandible", *American Journal of Diseases of Childhood*; 48; 541–547. Cited in Wagener, et al. 2002.

24. Wagener, S., Rayatt, S.S., Tatman, A.J., Gornall, P. and Slator, R. (2003) "Management of infants with Pierre Robin Sequence", *Cleft Palate Craniofacial Journal*; 20; 2; 180–185.

25. Lightwood, R. and Brimblecombe, F.S.W. (1963) Donald Paterson's *SICK CHILDREN, Diagnosis and Treatment*, chapter 13, Disorders of the Respiratory System, Cassell, London. 224–225.

26. Bromley, D and Burston, W.R. (1966) "The Pierre Robin Syndrome", *Nursing Times*; 62; 52; 1717–1720.

27. Matthews, D.N. (1957) Plastic Surgery in Moncrieff, A. and Norman, A.P. A *Textbook on the Nursing and Diseases of Sick Children*, H.K. Lewis & Co. Ltd, London.

28. Lost Hospitals of London (alphabetical list) accessed at ezitis-myzen.co.uk hammersmith html

29. Wikipedia – Joe Loss, accessed March 2021 from https://en.wikipedia.org/wiki/Joe_Loss

30. Levinson, H. (2011) "The strange and curious history of lobectomy", BBC News, 8 November 10.48.

31. Royal College of Surgeons – accessed July 2020, "Lives of the Fellows – Waterston, David James" (1910–1985).

32. Graham, G. (1995) "Obituaries: Richard Bonham-Carter", *Independent*, Monday 20 February 1995 01.02.

33. Gosh.nhs.uk, "Heart and Lung Breakthrough Guide", accessed March 2020 at www.gosh.nhs.uk

34. Ashcraft, K.W. (1987) "Obituary, Eoin Aberdeen, June 15, 1923 to March 24, 1986", *Journal of Paediatric Surgery*; 22; 3; 301.

35. Wikipedia "Mustard procedure". Accessed March 2020 at: en.wikipedia.org/wiki/Mustard_procedure

36. Hacket, K. (2017) "Leaving a lasting Legacy", *Nursing Children and Young People*, 29; 8; 19.

37. Gibson, T. (1697) "The Anatomy of the Humane Bodies Epitomized", Awnsham and Churchill, London England, (Ed. 5), cited in Spitz, L. (1996) "Esophageal Atresia: Past, Present, and Future", *Journal of Paediatric Surgery*, Vol 31; 1; 19-26.

38. Spitz, L. (1996) "Esophageal Atresia: Past, Present, and Future", *Journal of paediatric Surgery*; 31; 1; 19-25.

39. Spitz, L. (2006) "Esophageal Atresia: Lessons I have Learned in a 40-year experience", *Journal of Paediatric Surgery*; 41; 1635–1640, from Elsevier Inc.

40. Aberdeen, E. (1964) "Oesophageal Atresia and Tracheo-oesophageal Fistula", *Nursing Times*; 60; 789–791.

41. Sherman, C.D. and Waterston, D. (1957) "Oesophageal Reconstruction in Children using Intrathoracic Colon", *Archives of Diseases in Childhood*, downloaded from: http://adc.bmj.com on 14 July 2020.

42. Waterston, D.J., Bonham Carter, R.E. and Aberdeen, E. (1962) "Oesophageal Atresia: Tracheo-Oesophageal Fistula – A Study of Survival in 218 Infants", *The Lancet*; 1; 819-822.

43. Esenlik, E. (2015) "Presurgical Infant Orthopaedics for Cleft Lip and Palate: A Review", *Journal of Surgery*, 11 (1); 313–318.

44. Rosenstein, W.S. (1963) "Early Orthodontic Procedures for Cleft Lip and Palate Individuals", *The Angle Orthodontist*, Vol. XXX111; no. 2; 127–137.

45. Lienhard, J.H. (accessed, April 2020) "Engines of Our Ingenuity, 'Holter's Brain Drain', a lecture by Neurosurgeon Peyman Pakzaban", accessed at https://uh.edu/engines/epi2582.htm

46. McKissock, W. (1957) "Neurosurgery" from Moncrieff, A. and Norman, A.P. *A Textbook on the Nursing and Diseases of Sick Children*, H.K. Lewis & Co. Ltd, London.

47. Mazur, J.M. (2005) Casey Memorial Lectureship: "Adult consequences of Spina Bifida" from 49th Annual Meeting of the Society for Research into Hydrocephalus and Spina Bifida, Barcelona, Spain 29 June – 2 July 2005. Published in Cerebrospinal Fluid 2005; 2 (1): s44.

48. Boockvar, J.A., Loudon, W. and Sutton, L.N. (2001) "Development of the Spitz-Holter valve in Philadelphia", *Journal of Neurosurgery*, 95 (1)

49. Wikipedia "Queen Mary's Hospital, Roehampton". Accessed April 2020 at: en.wikipedia.org/Queen_Mary%27s_Hospital,_Roehampton

50. Starns, P. (1997) "Military Influence on the British Civilian Nursing Profession 1939 – 1969", Phd. Dissertation for the University of Bristol, Ref.1: page 92; Refs:2 & 3 page 38. Accessed April 2020 from: http://research-information.bristol.ac.uk

51. Encel, S. (1968) "Armed Forces and Society", Netherlands p.138, cited in Starns, P. (1997) "Military Influence on the British Civilian Nursing Profession 1939–1969", page 38.

52. II Kings 920. Holy Bible. Authorised Version, Oxford University Press.

53. Stanford, J. (1966) *Cathy Come Home*, BBC Television play. Accessed October 2021 from: en.wikipedia.org/wiki/Cathy_Come_Home

54. Dewer, H.A. (1978) "The hospital nurse after Salmon and Briggs" from The state of British medicine, *Journal of the Royal Society of Medicine*. Vol 71; 399–400.

55. Gray, J. (1990) "Staying put", *Nursing Standard*, 4; 29; 54.

56. Ivac (Last revised 2013), accessed April 2020, The Ivac legacy. The San Diego Technological Archive at: http://libraries.ucsd.edu/sdta

57. Dudrick, S.J. (1977) "The genesis of intravenous hyperalimentation". *Journal of parenteral and Enteral Nutrition 1 (1)*. Accessed April 2020 from: https://onlinelibrary.wiley.com

58. Sanchez, J.A. and Daly, J.M. (2010) "Stanley J Dudrick, MD, A Paradigm Shift". *The Archives of Surgery*; 145; 6; 512–514.

59. Dudrick, S.J., et al. (1968) "Long-term total parenteral nutrition with growth, development and positive nitrogen balance". *Surgery*, 64: 134–142.

60. Carlson, M. (2016) Medical research, Henry Heimlich Obituary, *Guardian*, 20 December 2016.

61. Gosh.nhs.uk, Breakthroughs in children's medicine pdf. Accessed September 2020 at www.gosh.nhs.uk

62. Gosh.nhs.uk – "Separating conjoined twins Safa and Marwa", accessed October 2020 at: https://www.gosh.nhs.uk/news/ seoarating-conjoined-twins-safa-and-marwa

63. Wikipedia (accessed September 2021) List of epidemics at: En.wikipedia.org/wiki/list_of_epidemics

64. Royal Brompton and Harefield, Our History Accessed at rbht.nhs. uk/about-us/our-history

65. Martin, V. (1981) "A burning issue – Preventing hypertrophic scarring", *Nursing Mirror* 153; 16; 32–34.

66. BBC Home On this day (21) 1979 Harrier crash kills three. Accessed October 2020.

67. Wisbech Cambridgeshire Community Archive Network, "Newspaper cutting reporting on an airplane crash in Ranmoth Road, Wisbech that occurred in 1979". Accessed 18/05/20.

68. Elidyr Communities Trust, "A Fantastic Place to Live and Learn". Accessed October 2020 from elidyrct.ac.uk

69. Martin, V. (1993) "Growing confidence". *Nursing Times*; 89; 48; 44–46.

GLOSSARY

A

Abscess – a swelling containing pus and located anywhere in the body.

Adenoids – a collection of tissue at the back of the nose used to trap germs which otherwise may cause infection.

Anaemia – a reduction in the quantity of the oxygen-carrying haemoglobin in the blood.

Anaesthetic (General) – inhaled agents used to depress the central nervous system to produce unconsciousness before a surgical procedure.

Anaesthetise – to induce unconsciousness prior to an operation.

Anaesthetist – a medically qualified doctor who administers an anaesthetic to induce unconsciousness in a patient.

Antibiotic – medication that destroys or inhibits the growth of bacteria or fungi that are sensitive to them.

Antihistamine – a drug that inhibits the effects of histamine, part of the body's defence system, particularly to reduce allergic reactions.

Appendix – a short tube with a blind end, at the junction of the large and small intestine or gut.

Aseptic technique – a healthcare procedure that excludes bacteria, fungi and viruses to minimise the risk of infection.

Aspiration pneumonia – when fluid enters the lungs causing them to become inflamed.

Asthma – a condition resulting in spasm of the tubes to the lungs, causing difficulty in breathing.

Atresia – absence or abnormal narrowing of a body opening.

Autoclave – an airtight steel vessel used for sterilising surgical instruments or dressings. It is similar to a pressure cooker, into which articles are placed and treated with steam at high pressure.

Auxiliary Nurse – a support worker who assists the trained nurses.

B

Bile – a fluid from the liver via the bile duct, which enables fats to be more easily digested.

Biopsy – the removal of a small piece of living tissue from an organ or part of the body for microscopic examination.

Bladder – the organ that stores urine.

Bleep – a device which makes a high-pitched sound to gain attention.

Bowel – part of the gut or intestine which extends from the stomach to the back passage.

C

Cannular – a hollow tube designed to insert into a body cavity such as the bladder or a blood vessel.

Cardiac – relating to or affecting the heart.

Cardiac arrest – when the heart suddenly stops pumping blood around the body.

Catheter – a tube for insertion into a narrow opening so that fluids may be introduced or removed.

Catheterisation – introduction of a catheter into the bladder to relieve obstruction to the outflow of urine.

Cheatle forceps – long forceps used to take dressings and instruments from autoclaved drums.

Cleft – an opening or a gap.

Coeliac disease – when the immune system attacks the lining of the small bowel after a person eats gluten.

Coma or Comatosed – a state of unrousable unconsciousness.

Congenital – a condition recognised at birth or that is believed to have been present since birth.

Consultant – a fully trained specialist in a branch of medicine or surgery who accepts total responsibility for patient care.

Crash team – an "on call" team of medical and nursing staff who attend emergency situations, mainly if a patient's heart stops and/or the patient stops breathing (the latter particularly in the case of a child).

Cross Chart – a book of competencies used by student nurses entitled "Record of practical instruction for the Certificate of Nursing Sick Children".

Curate – a cleric assisting a parish priest.

Cyst – a sac-like structure in the body containing fluid or gas.

Cystic Fibrosis – a hereditary disease causing a number of glands to discharge abnormally thick mucus into the body.

D

Dialysis – a process of filtering waste particles through a membrane.

Diocese – an area comprised of a number of parishes presided over by a bishop.

Drain – a device for removing fluid from a cavity or wound.

E

Eczema – inflammation of the outer layer of the skin causing itching and a red rash, often accompanied by blisters that weep and become crusted.

Enema – the insertion and removal of fluid into and out of the back passage.

E.N.T. – Ear Nose and Throat.

Ether – a colourless liquid, the fumes of which were inhaled as an anaesthetic.

F

Faeces – waste matter or bodily excretions.

Fallot's Tetralogy – a heart condition with which a baby may be born. Such a child has three problems, the narrowing of the main artery to the lungs, the enlargement of the chamber of the heart which pumps the blood to the lungs and a hole in the heart.

Fistula – an opening or an abnormal communication between two hollow organs.

Forceps – a pincer-like instrument designed to grasp an object.

G

Gaberdine mac – a waxed waterproof coat worn by nurses to cover their uniform.

Gall bladder – a sac which lies underneath the right-hand part (lobe) of the liver and stores bile.

Gastric – relating to the stomach.

Gastrostomy – a surgical operation in which an opening is made through the abdominal wall into the stomach. It is usually performed to allow food and fluid to be poured directly into the stomach when swallowing is difficult or impossible.

Genetic coding – the information carried by the DNA (our hereditary material).

Geriatric – a branch of medicine concerned with the treatment of diseases that occur in old age.

Glue ear – when the empty part of the middle ear fills with fluid, causing hearing loss.

Great Arteries – the arteries that carry blood away from the heart.

H

Haemodialysis – a technique of removing waste materials from the blood in kidney failure by dialysis.

Haemoglobin – a substance contained within red blood cells responsible for their colour and the transportation of oxygen within the body.

Haemolytic streptococcal bacteria – an infection that has the ability to destroy red blood cells.

Hernia – the protrusion of an organ or tissue out of the body cavity in which it lies.

Hormone – a substance produced in one part of the body which passes into the bloodstream and is carried to other organs or tissue where it acts to modify their structure or function.

Hycolin – a disinfectant.

Hydrocephalus – an abnormal amount of fluid within the ventricles of the brain.

I

Immune system – mechanism by which the body resists infection.

Immunity – the body's ability to resist infection.

Immunosuppressant drug – a drug that reduces the body's resistance to fight infection.

Incubator – a transparent container for keeping premature babies in controlled conditions to help control their body temperatures and protect them from infections.

Infection – invasion of the body by harmful organisms e.g. bacteria, fungi or viruses.

Infusion – a slow injection of fluid into a vein.

Intramuscular injection – an injection into a muscle.

Intravenous – into or within a vein.

Intubate – the putting of a tube into the patient's throat to give an anaesthetic or to aid the expansion of their lungs.

J

Jaundice – a yellowing of the skin and/or whites of the eyes indicating excess bilirubin (a bile pigment) in the blood. It is caused by either excessive destruction of the red cells in the blood, or problems with the liver.

K

Kardex – a file of nursing records.

Kidney dish – a stainless steel kidney shaped dish.

L

Laceration – a tear in the flesh producing a wound with irregular edges.

Last offices – care given to a body after death.

Lesion – an abnormal change in tissue.

Leukaemia (including acute Lymphoblastic Leukaemia) – a group of malignant diseases in which the bone marrow and other blood forming organs produce increased numbers of white blood cells. The overproduction of these cells, which are in an immature or abnormal form, suppress the production of normal blood cells.

M

Malignant – describing a tumour which invades and destroys the tissue in which it originates.

Malnutrition – a condition caused by eating too little food, inappropriate food or a failure to digest what is eaten.

Matins – a morning prayer service.

Mezzanine floor – an intermediate floor. In this case, the floor between the ground and first floor.

Microbiology department – a department that identifies organisms that cause disease and identifies ways of treating them.

Mumps – a viral infection typified by swelling of the glands around the jaw.

N

Nebuliser – an instrument used for applying a liquid in the form of a fine spray.

Neonate – an infant just born or in the first four weeks of life.

Nits – the empty egg cases from which head lice hatch.

O

Obstetrics – the branch of medicine concerned with the care of women during pregnancy, childbirth and a period of about six weeks following the birth.

Oesophageal Artesia (O.A.) – a blind end to the tube that should take food from the throat to the stomach.

Oesophagostomy – a surgical operation by which the oesophagus is diverted to open on to the neck.

Oesophagus – a muscular tube at the back of the throat that takes food to the stomach.

Ophthalmic surgery – surgery relating to the eye.

Oral surgery – surgery relating to the mouth.

Orthodontics – the art and science of correcting misplaced teeth using dental appliances.

Orthopaedic – the science or practice of correcting deformities or damage to bones and joints of the body.

P

Paediatrics – the general medicine of childhood.

Palate – the roof of the mouth.

Peritoneal Cavity – the space that surrounds the wall of the abdomen and protects the abdominal organs.

Peritoneal dialysis – using the lining of the abdomen to filter waste material and water from the bloodstream in kidney failure.

Physician – a registered medical practitioner who specialises in the diagnosis and treatment of disease by other than surgical means.

Physiotherapist – a health practitioner qualified to treat injury, disease or deformity using exercise, massage or heat treatment.

PICU – Paediatric Intensive Care Unit.

Plaster of Paris – a preparation of gypsum (calcium sulphate) that sets hard when water is added. It is used in orthopaedics for preparing a rigid casing to support a limb.

Premedication – a drug given to a patient before an operation which calms the patient down and dries up the secretions of the lungs (which otherwise might be inhaled during the anaesthetic).

Psychiatrist – a medically qualified physician who specialises in the study and treatment of mental disorders.

Psychologist (Clinical Psychologist)– someone who studies the human mind, human emotions and behaviour, and how situations have an effect on people

R

Registrar – an experienced physician or surgeon working with a consultant, responsible for the care of patients and assisted by junior doctors whom he/she instructs.

Renal – relating to or affecting the kidneys.

Respiratory arrest – when a patient stops breathing or is breathing ineffectively.

Resuscitation – the process to correct a lack of breathing or heartbeat in an acutely ill patient.

RSCN – Registered Sick Children's Nurse qualification.

S

Sedate – to produce a restful state of mind by the use of drugs (sedatives).

Sham feeding – a feed given to babies who cannot feed normally, to enable them to experience being fed by mouth and learn to develop normal sucking and swallowing co-ordination.

Shroud – a sheet or wrapping for a patient who has died.

Sluice – a room used for the hygienic disposal of waste.

Soft palate – the back part of the roof of the mouth consisting mainly of muscle.

"Specialling" – describes an experienced nurse giving one-to-one care to a patient.

SRN – State Registered Nurse.

Status Asthmaticus – an attack of asthma, lasting more than 24 hours, that causes great distress. It carries a risk of death from respiratory failure or exhaustion.

Strings cap – a distinctive cap, used to be worn by Great Ormond Street Hospital nurses in their final year of training and as a staff nurse.

Supernummerary tooth – a tooth growing outside the gum area.

Suppository – a medicinal preparation in solid form suitable for insertion into the back passage.

Syndrome – a combination of symptoms that form a distinct definition of a condition.

T

Tetanus – a bacterial infection which affects the nervous system.

Theology – a study of the nature of God and religious belief.

Tissue – the material consisting of cells, from which we are made.

Toxins – poisons produced by living organisms.

Tracheo-oesophageal fistula – an abnormal opening between the windpipe (trachea) and the food pipe (oesophagus).

Tracheostomy – an opening made in the front of the neck, where a tube is inserted into the wind pipe to assist with breathing.

Traction – the application of a pulling force with weights, ropes and pullies to ensure a broken bone is kept in the correct position during the early stages of healing.

Transposition of the Great Arteries – a condition where the two main blood vessels of the heart, the pulmonary artery (which takes blood to the lungs) and the aorta (which takes blood to the body) are transposed (or swapped over).

U

Underwater seal drain – a chest drain, draining the chest cavity of air, blood or fluid through a water seal to restore negative pressure.

Urine – fluid excreted by the kidneys and stored in the bladder, which contains many of the body's waste products.

Urology – a branch of medicine concerned with the study of the urinary tract.

V

Vaccine – a preparation given to stimulate the body to produce antibodies and an immunity against a specific or a number of diseases.

VAD – Voluntary Aid Detachment nurse – volunteer civilians who provided care for military personnel wounded during World Wars I and II.

Venous line – tube into a vein.

Ventilator – a machine to artificially oxygenate the blood in the lungs.

Ventricles – one of the four fluid-filled cavities of the brain, or one of the two lower chambers of the heart.

X

X-ray – electromagnetic radiation of extremely low wavelength, which can create a picture of the inside of the body.

Main reference used: *Concise Medical Dictionary* (1981) Editor Martin, E.D. Oxford University Press Medical Publications.

ACKNOWLEDGEMENTS

I would like to thank: Nicholas Baldwin Archivist, Great Ormond Street NHS Foundation Trust, for his interest in my book and his research, John Curtis for his advice on publishing, Sophie Duffy for developing my text and leaving less to the imagination, Carol Edwards (née Pearson) for sharing her memories and helping to jog mine, Professor David Hannay for checking my glossary, Patricia for her enthusiasm for this book and her memories of GOSH, William Robson for his valuable help with photographs, Adelaide Tunstill, many years a Sister on the Thoracic Unit at Great Ormond Street, for her helpful insights,

The past patients and their families who have recalled their experiences and sent me contributions and many other friends who have shared their memories and given me encouragement.

A special thanks goes to the Information Specialists from the Royal College of Nursing Scotland library, Emma Taylor and Abigail Kleboe, for their tireless literature searches and for accessing many of my references. Without them I would not have been able to complete a number of my patient studies in this book.

A final thank you goes to Ajda Vucicevic for commissioning me to write this book.